Adaptogens

Adaptogens

A Directory of Over 50 Healing
Herbs for Energy, Stress Relief,
Beauty, and Overall Well-Being

Melissa Petitto, R. D.

chartwell
books

Quarto

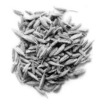

This edition published in 2022 by Chartwell Books,
an imprint of The Quarto Group
142 West 36th Street, 4th Floor
New York, NY 10018 USA
T (212) 779-4972 F (212) 779-6058
www.Quarto.com

First published in 2020 by Chartwell Books,
an imprint of The Quarto Group
142 West 36th Street, 4th Floor
New York, NY 10018 USA
T (212) 779-4972 F (212) 779-6058
www.Quarto.com

10 9 8 7 6 5 4 3 2

ISBN: 978-0-7858-4190-6

Library of Congress Cataloging-in-Publication
Data available upon request.

Chartwell titles are also available at discount for
retail, wholesale, promotional, and bulk purchase. For
details, contact the Special Sales Manager by email
at specialsales@quarto.com or by mail at The Quarto
Group, Attn: Special Sales Manager, 100 Cummings
Center Suite 265D, Beverly, MA 01915, USA.

Publisher: Wendy Friedman
Editorial Director: Betina Cochran
Senior Design Manager: Michael Caputo
Editor: Jennifer Kushnier
Interior Design: Tara Long
Cover Design: Sue Boylan

Printed in China

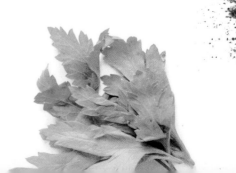

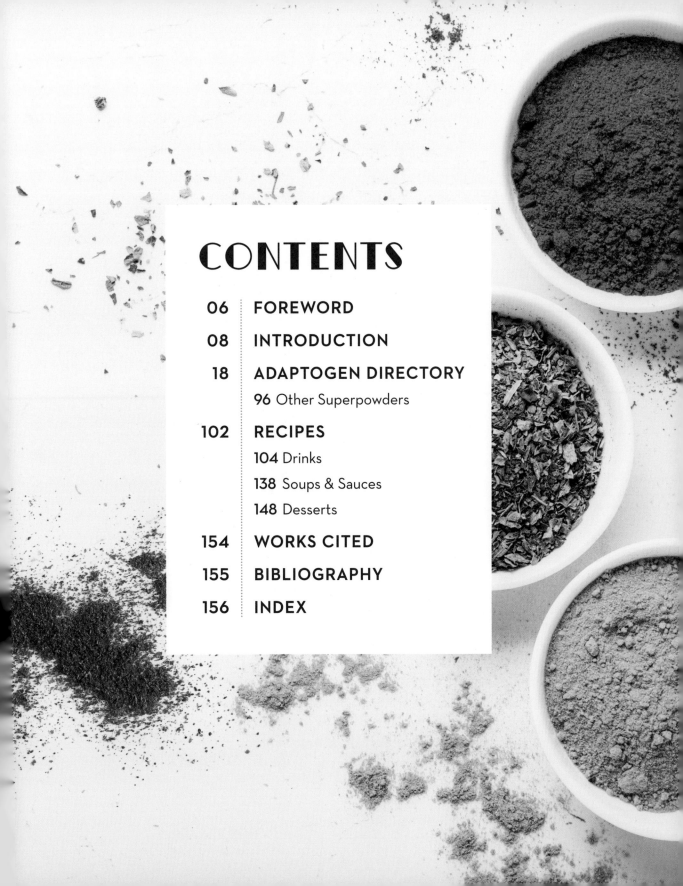

CONTENTS

FOREWORD

Walk in a forest, smell the flowers, feel the thunderous clap of waves hitting the beach; nature in all its beauty can change the way we feel in an instant. At one moment meditative and calming, at other times refreshing and invigorating. Our sense of wellness is intimately connected to our environment.

In fact, our hectic modern life, with its increased light, noise, and environmental pollution, is often devoid of nature's rejuvenating and restorative benefits. The way we live is instead associated with a higher incidence of depression, anxiety, allergies, and autoimmune disease.

Where Western medicine lacks the tools, ancient healing traditions and naturopathic medicine may provide the answers we need to preserve wellness in this increasingly demanding environment. Healers across cultures have recognized that the mind and body are intricately intertwined and should be seen as one. Chinese medicine, natural medicine, and Ayurveda use plants to address patterns that emerge when our health is out of balance. Plants have been prescribed as cooling, such as peppermint extract to reduce the fever and heat associated with colds and the flu. Milk thistle is used for people with a yellow complexion associated with liver conditions. We now know that the active components in peppermint are flavonoids, and milk thistle contains silymarins. Over the last couple of decades, functional nutritional medicine has revealed the mechanisms by which these plants' powerful phytonutrients reduce inflammation, limit oxidative stress, and balance the microbiome. As a naturopathic doctor, I am fascinated by how the ancient traditional use of plants can now be understood through the lens of biochemistry.

A patient walked into my office a couple of months ago. He was a salesman suffering from recurring colds, fatigue, depression, and digestive upset. He'd been working long hours for many years. He ate poorly, often skipping meals, eating fast food, and consuming heavy meals late at night. A recent visit to his primary physician showed slightly elevated cholesterol, but no recommendations were made. It was clear that, at the heart of it all, he was no longer able to adapt to the demands of his lifestyle. This was expressed physically with a weakening immune system and cardiovascular and mental-emotional imbalance.

The answer was a program that included adaptogenic herbs such as ashwagandha and rhodiola rosea. I suggested that he take prebiotic baobab fruit powder, which is derived from the baobab, known as the African tree of life. It's a substance rich in vitamin C, antioxidants, and prebiotic fiber. In addition, I prescribed a plant-based diet and a daily meditative practice. Only two weeks later, the shifts in his condition were remarkable: he was able to sleep and his digestion was better.

More than ever, we need nature to guide us in balancing the increased demands of this fast-moving world. In this book, Melissa Petitto, R.D., offers a great overview of adaptogens—their traditional uses, their modern applications, and how they can be safely and creatively included in your everyday health routine.

Dr. Luc Maes, N.D.
Director, The Maes Center for Natural Health Care, Santa Barbara
Founder KAIBAE, The Lost Crops Company

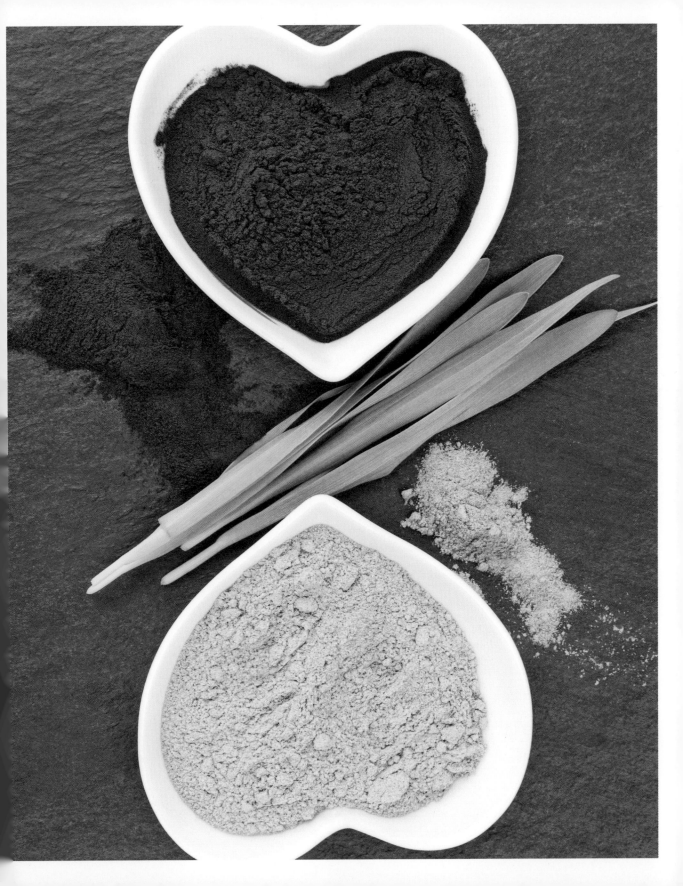

INTRODUCTION

Welcome to the ancient world of herbal healing. It's ancient because the practice of using plants for health, healing, and wellness has been in place for millennia. And by "herbal," I'm not talking about what you might be growing in your garden. Rather, I mean everything from herbs, beans, and mushrooms to roots and fruit, bark and flowers, leaves and stems, even pollen and pearls. While some of these natural substances we ingest in their natural form, others we turn into extracts, tinctures, teas, and powders. (And in this book, we'll put them to delicious use with simple recipes, whether it's for easing grief or PMS, or boosting muscle strength or gut health.)

In the pages that follow, we'll explore 38 "intelligent plants," known as adaptogens, and their wealth of health benefits, including the 2000-year-old mushroom called the "elixir of immortality" and the fruit Genghis Khan used to power his army. We'll find out which substances can cure hangovers, achieve a youthful appearance, remedy gray hairs, or alleviate "new-mom brain"—including dosages, warnings, and other benefits in the body. So let's dive into this vast world of plant-based wellness by starting at the beginning, with Ayurveda and Traditional Chinese Medicine.

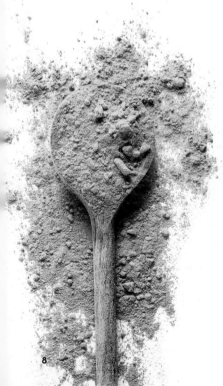

AYURVEDA AND TRADITIONAL CHINESE MEDICINE

Ayurveda is a traditional Hindu system of medicine that originated over five thousand years ago and was verbally passed down from masters until it was finally written down. It is based on the belief that we balance our bodily systems through herbal treatment, diet, and yogic breathing. In Sanskrit, *ayurveda* can be translated as "the science of life."

The system as a whole places great emphasis on prevention, as opposed to Western medicine's focus on treatment after the fact. This means that Ayurveda fosters a balance in our minds and bodies, with a focus on what we put into our bodies, what herbs we ingest, and the lifestyle we follow. Ayurveda also believes that each person has a unique configuration of energy; an individual combination of physical, mental, and emotional characteristics that makes each person a whole unique individual.

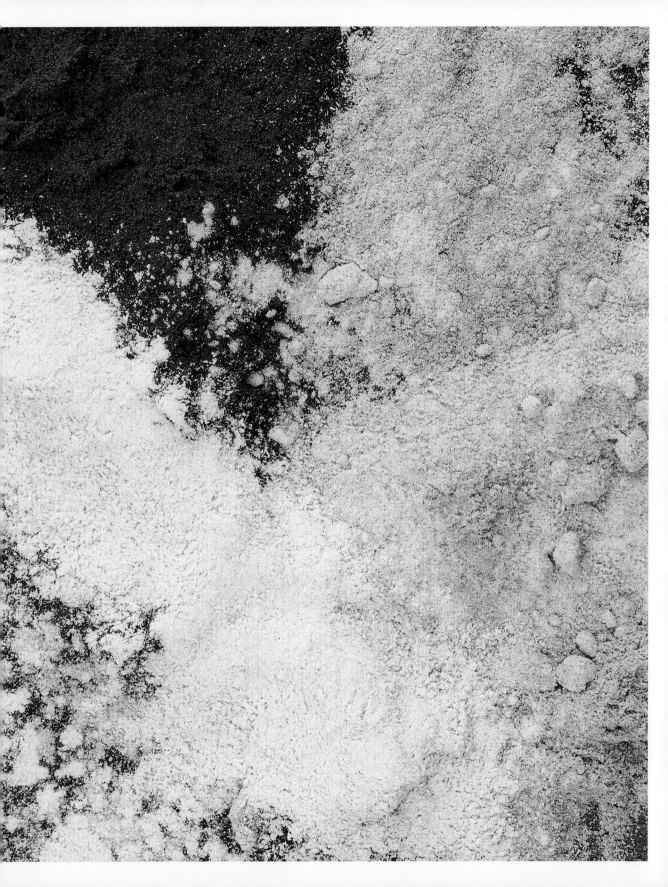

What I love most about Ayurveda is this: balance is the natural order, imbalance is disorder. Health is order, disease is disorder. When you understand your own body, you can reestablish order with diet, lifestyle, and herbs. Ayurveda further breaks down our body types into doshas: Vata, Pitta, and Kapha. There are online quizzes to help you determine your body type, which includes your primary and subordinate dosha. A truly balanced body is one where the three doshas are in balance, something that the right diet, lifestyle, and herbs can help. Enter the adaptogenic herbs in Ayurveda. Of these varieties, rasayana herbs in Ayurveda were shown to increase energy, while also promoting youthfulness and increasing resistance to disease; these have come to be known today as adaptogens.

Like Ayurveda, Traditional Chinese Medicine (TCM) focuses on the well-being of the entire person (unlike Western medicine, which focuses mainly on treating the disease alone). Chinese medicine includes, but is not limited to, the fields of acupuncture, acupressure, herbs, meditation, and exercise.

With its emphasis on balance, harmony, and energy, there are two central foci in TCM. The first focus of Chinese medicine is qi, the vital energy that flows along meridians through our bodies and keeps a person's spiritual, emotional, mental, and physical health in balance. This qi runs throughout our bodies and can become "stuck" with illness and dis-ease (meaning lack of balance and harmony in the body). With the addition of acupuncture, herbs, meditation, and exercise, TCM helps promote and maintain the flow of qi. Yin and yang form the second central idea of TCM. These two opposites describe what makes up qi.

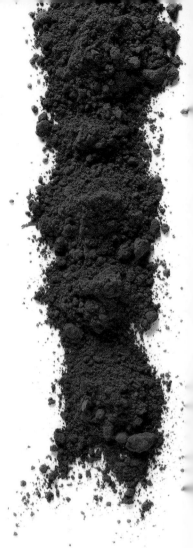

YIN
dark, night, spirit, negative, feminine

YANG
light, day, form, positive, male

Balance is everything. For every little bit of darkness there is light, and for every bit of femininity, there is masculinity. When we are balanced in yin and yang, our qi flows and we are healthy. In TCM, herbs are grouped into categories: the major one contains what are considered the "superior" herbs, which are respected for their tonic and synchronizing power on our complete health, what we would now call adaptogens.

WHAT ARE ADAPTOGENS?

While the term *adaptogens* is getting a lot of buzz in the wellness community right now, this classification of "intelligent plants" is not new. As we've seen, the practice of using herbs for wellness dates back to ancient Chinese and Ayurvedic medicine. But the word itself was coined in 1947 by a Soviet doctor and scientist, Nikolai V. Lazarev. During World War II, Russian scientists were instructed to find or create substances that could enhance the performance and stamina of the country's athletes and military.

Twenty years later, in 1968, Dr. Israel I. Brekhman and Dr. I. V. Dardymov revised the definition of an adaptogen and created the standards that we use today. They defined a class of mushrooms and herbs that must have three properties:

1 Be nontoxic to the body's physiological functions

2 Offer widespread support, including physical, chemical, and biological

3 Help bring the body back into equilibrium

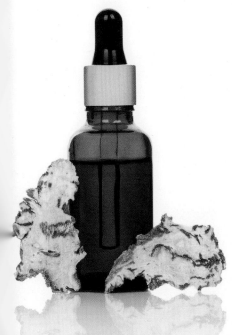

ALWAYS SEE THE BIGGER PICTURE

While these herbs and mushrooms can offer miraculous results, we need to remember that they are not a quick—or even the sole—solution to the stress of modern times. Rather, they provide an incredible addition to our lives for increasing our biological resilience and intensifying cell communication. Stress in our time is constant and comes in the form of being overscheduled, feeling stretched too thin, being constantly available to others through our cell phones and on social media: these conditions create a perfect storm for adrenal fatigue or simply being burned out. This is often the root cause of our dis-ease.

Plants, no matter how powerful they are, are not a substitute for getting enough sleep, eating whole, unprocessed foods, exercising, spending time in nature, or other healthy pursuits like taking care of our hearts through meaningful, loving relationships. All of these are crucial for maintaining the balance of our minds, bodies, and spirits. Adaptogens are intelligent plants that we can add to this healthy mix.

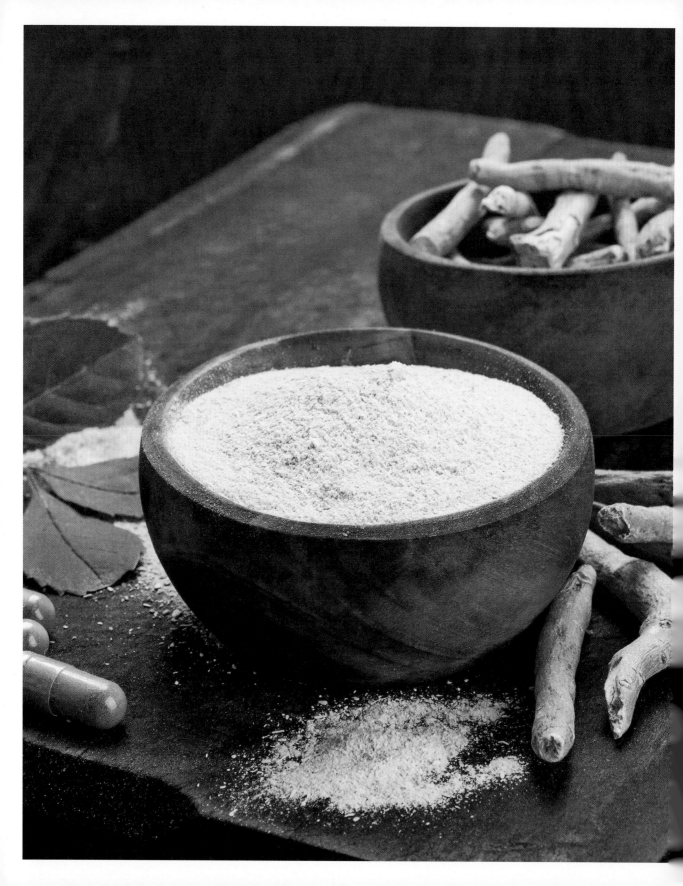

INTELLIGENT PLANTS

Adaptogenic plants are numerous and vary in their intelligent abilities to help raise our bodies' resistance to environmental toxin exposure, emotional trauma, and mental fatigue stressors. They all have one thing in common, though: their ability to help the body better *adapt* to stress. Cortisol, the stress and aging hormone, is the root cause of many of our ailments. Adaptogens target and support our adrenals, the glands that handle hormonal response to stress and help us manage our anxiety and fatigue. Beyond this, they have an uncanny, chameleon-like ability to adapt to our bodies' specific needs and restore homeostasis (balance). When we add adaptogens to our daily routine, they help minimize the effects of stress hormones and help the body respond to stress in a healthier way.

Adding these intelligent plants in your life could lead to many amazing results, including:

- Enhancing immunity
- Guarding against disease
- Increasing energy
- Easing symptoms of depression and anxiety
- Balancing moods

- Supporting cognitive abilities
- Minimizing fatigue
- Improving focus
- Bringing balance back to metabolic processes
- Boosting libido

- Reducing cravings for sugar, carbohydrates, and processed foods
- Sensing harmony
- Elevating consciousness
- Promoting overall well-being

Within the classification of adaptogens there are two basic types. Some are known to stimulate the body, improve mental performance, and increase physical stamina. Examples include eleuthero, rhodiola rosea, maca, and Asian ginseng. Those that help soothe the adrenals by relaxing the body fall into another classification; these include the reishi mushroom, holy basil, and ashwagandha.

STRESS AND THE BODY

Let's take a closer look at what the adrenal glands are and how they handle stressors.

The adrenal glands are part of the endocrine system, which also includes the thyroid and reproductive organs. The adrenal glands produce hormones, such as adrenaline and cortisol. These hormones help to regulate heart rate, blood pressure, the way the body uses food, the levels of minerals in the body, as well as how we react to stressors throughout the day.

Let's break this down further to understand what actually happens when we feel stress. Our bodies naturally seek homeostasis, but when we look at all the stressors in our everyday life, we find many sources for imbalance.

When we encounter a major stressor, our adrenals release cortisol and adrenaline, preparing us to take on whatever it is that we need to fight. Our heart rate and blood sugar rise, getting us ready for fight or flight. After the stressor passes, we return to normal. The problem lies in the fact that we often live in a state of chronic stress, which means we have incredibly high levels of cortisol, pumping through us all the time. This can lead to thyroid problems, depression, anxiety, weight gain, mood swings, and sleep problems.

TO REITERATE: Healthy habits like getting good sleep, eating whole, unprocessed foods, engaging in regular exercise, spending time in nature, practicing self-care, and ingesting powerful plants may help control the problem.caused by chronic stress.

Sleep and how I react to stressful situations remain two of the most difficult and important health factors I experience in my own life. Sleep is *a lot* different from what I had expected before I became a mother. Sleep deprivation is something that we as parents are used to, but that doesn't mean we aren't subject to intense mood-altering effects all the same. Moodiness, sluggishness, strange and disrupted eating habits, feeling uninspired, reacting in a less-than-desired way—all of these are par for the course when our sleep is less than optimal.

What if, by adding intelligent plants and mushrooms into our daily lives, we could help change the way we react to situations? Could we allow our bodies to naturally calm down at night? Help turn off our minds and relax? Give us non-jittery, clean energy? Improve the way our body's adrenals function—to let them do the job they were *designed* to do—and help us deal with the daily stressors of everyday life? Adaptogens can offer a new kind of well-being: they are an excellent addition to help us be our best selves.

LET'S TALK ABOUT WHOLE FOODS

Let's face it: our current food system gives us less time to feed ourselves optimally. The soil in which our food is grown is depleted of nutrients because of our current farming techniques. Our bodies are stressed beyond belief, which in turn throws our digestion off. With this in mind, I think we could all benefit from a little extra ancient-herbal support.

We all know that consuming a varied diet of whole, unprocessed plants is optimal for gaining the vitamins, nutrients, and unique phytonutrients that each plant contains. Adaptogenic powders work to enhance the benefits contained in plants. As it turns out, the best powders are also made of real, whole foods that are simply dried and turned into superpowders (you'll get the most benefit from the least processed ones, so it's important to look for powders without preservatives or additives).

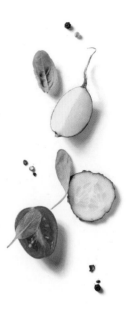

WHAT ABOUT SAFETY?

Adaptogenic plants are, by definition, safe and nontoxic. Even with this in mind, it is important to remember that too much of a good thing can be detrimental. You could have an allergic reaction or be highly sensitive to one of the plants, or you could have an adverse reaction with a medication. For this reason, it's always best to consult with a physician before adding these plants to your diet.

You can consult with a Traditional Chinese Medicine doctor, a naturopath, or a Western physician as long as they are a trusted professional. Some plants are not safe for pregnant women or those taking immunosuppressant drugs. Once you've consulted with a specialist you trust, you'll be ready to begin your incredible healing journey!

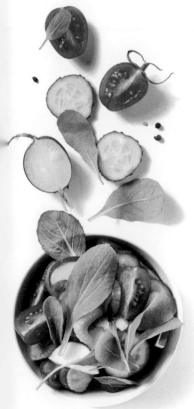

HOW LONG DO BENEFITS TAKE TO APPEAR?

These intelligent plants tend to work best when taken for a period of 6 to 8 weeks; if you don't see results immediately, don't lose patience until you've put in the full time. Adaptogens are meant to adapt with our lives. We don't maintain the same stress levels, lifestyle, or health challenges throughout life, so an adaptogen that works great in one stage of life might not help you in another. Think back to Ayurveda: each person has a different energy configuration, a combination of physical, mental, and emotional characteristics that make each individual unique. That means each person needs to find his or her own unique balance of these ancient healing plants.

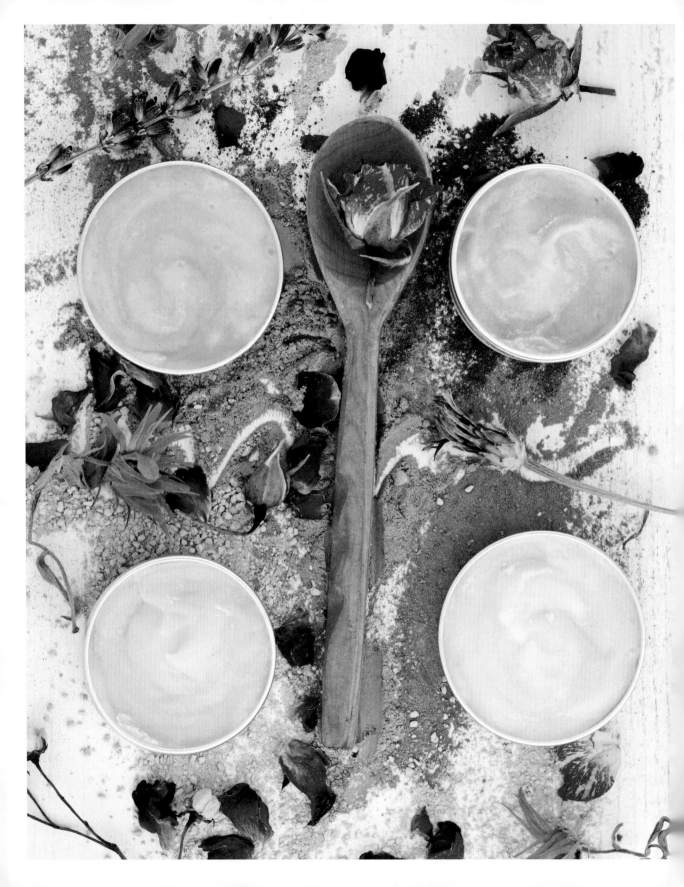

Here are some guidelines to help you begin your journey into wellness:

- Start with a single plant or herb to see how your body reacts. You may find the effects are too intense or discover that you are allergic to it.

- Once you know how your body responds to various herbs in isolation, pre-made blends are an incredible way to find true homeostasis in the body.

- Log any symptoms (or their absence) to track your progress. Be sure to switch up your intake if you feel something has changed.

- Taking a break from these plants can be beneficial. One day a week, one week a month, or one month a year is recommended.

- Adaptogens like to be rotated: switch them up every couple of months.

- Some herbals are great for children, but talk to your children's doctor before adding any to their diet.

- While you should always ask your doctor about incorporating anything into your routine when you're pregnant, some herbs can be amazing for milk supply when breastfeeding.

THOUGHTS ON HERBALISTS

Herbalists can achieve amazing results. They look at the outer self—the eyes, ears, and hands—but they also look below the surface, to the inner self—the mind, heart, and spirit. Herbalists peer into the point where our rational-self and our creative-self come together, a meeting that constitutes the true essence of who we are.

Herbalists believe that the mind cannot provide true healing by itself: it must be aided by the body and the wisdom of the heart. With that combination, there's a better chance of finding homeostasis and healing the whole self. Ancient healing herbs, when added to a healthy routine, have the power to aid in the prevention of stress-related diseases holistically and become a part of a wholistic approach to our well-being.

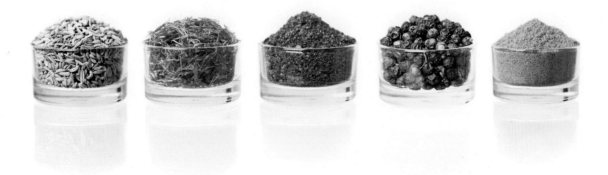

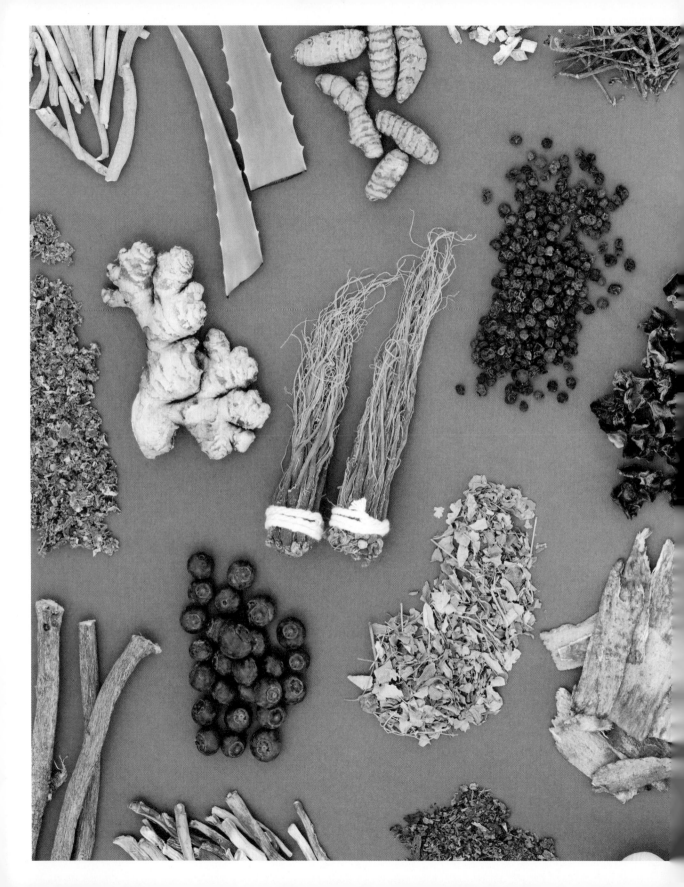

ADAPTOGEN DIRECTORY

Organized in alphabetical order by Latin name, this directory will help you navigate through various healing plants to find the best ones for your ailments or health goals. The icons below are included with each entry. The ones that are highlighted represent the greatest benefits you'll experience with each one.

STRESS REDUCTION

Lower cortisol, a stressor free system, and a happier you.

EXAMPLE: Asian ginseng improves your mental performance while reducing stress

SKIN

Free radical fighting, skin soothing, glowing skin.

EXAMPLE: Maca can help increase collagen synthesis in the skin and act as a protectant against the sun.

DIGESTION

Supports the gut biome, regularity, and maintaining a healthy gut.

EXAMPLE: Baobab is a prebiotic that feeds the friendly bacteria we need to maintain a healthy gut.

MENTAL CLARITY

Increases working concentration, memory, mental fatigue and focus.

EXAMPLE: Ashitaba has been shown to have anti-inflammatory effects which we now know helps reduce brain fog and enhance focus and clarity.

IMMUNITY BOOSTS

Aid in supporting and balancing the endocrine system.

EXAMPLE: Reishi contains beta-D glucan, which aids in boosting and enhancing the immune system while also reducing swelling with its anti-inflammatory properties.

ENERGY LEVELS

Increases energy, vitality, and fortitude.

EXAMPLE: Ashwagandha has an uncanny ability to support normal energy levels and regulate sleep patterns.

BAOBAB
ADANSONIA

HISTORY

This native African tree, also known as the "Tree of Life," is not only one of the most beautiful in nature, but it is one of the oldest. Some are said to be five thousand years old. They are seen as a symbol of life and positivity thriving in a terrain where little else can flourish. The tree may be one of the best known in the world, making appearances in *Avatar* and Disney's *The Lion King*, as well as my favorite book, *Le Petit Prince* by Antoine de Saint-Exupéry.

The fruit of the baobab is less well known, even though it's one of the most nutrient-dense foods in the world. Unique in nature, the fruit dries naturally while on its branch, taking six months to mature into a hard coconut-like pod. These dried pods are then harvested, deseeded, and sifted to produce a fine fruit powder. This fruit powder has been used as a food and as a natural source of health and beauty for centuries. Traditionally, the leaves, bark, and seeds are applied to treat malaria, microbial infections, fever, tuberculosis, dysentery, anemia, and diarrhea.

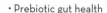

- Prebiotic gut health
- Lowers/controls blood sugar
- Alkalizer
- Electrolyte

DOSAGE

Take dried fruit, 1 to 2 teaspoons, up to two times a day.

BENEFITS

Baobab is the perfect prebiotic, an incredible aid in gut health. Probiotics took the wellness world by storm some years ago, but watch out for the *prebiotic*! It offers fuel for those gut-friendly bacteria we need to maintain a healthy gut. It has also been found to protect our immune function by protecting against illness, infections, and diseases.

Baobab is a natural energy source, reducing feelings of tiredness and fatigue. It supports skin health, stimulating the production of collagen and fighting the signs of aging. This well-rounded powder is a great source of vitamin C, calcium, phosphorus, magnesium, zinc, dietary fiber, potassium, lysine, protein, and lipids.

SAFETY

Ingesting baobab has no known adverse effects. Always consult your physician before adding it to your routine.

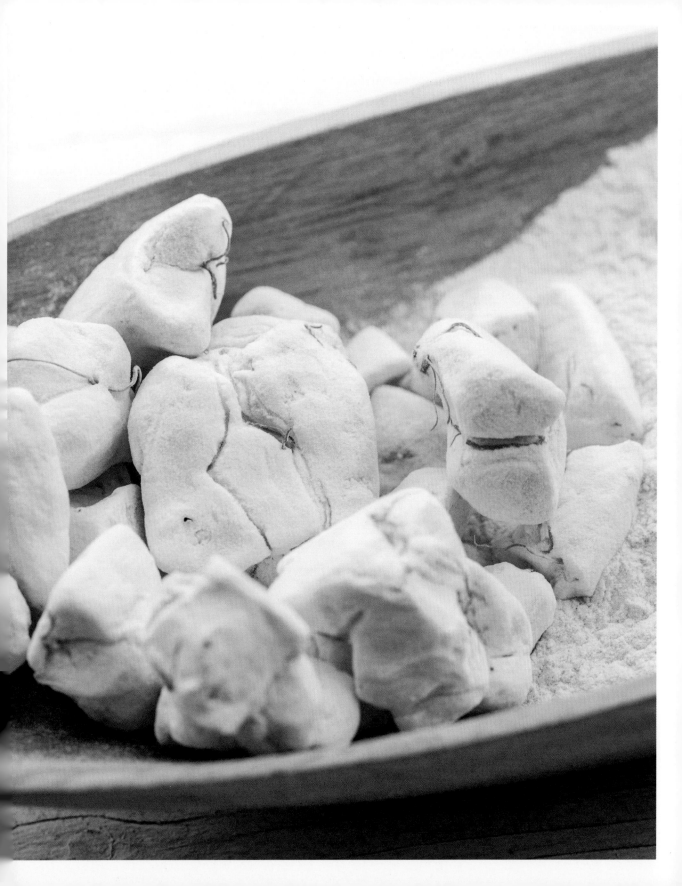

HIMEMATSUTAKE
(GOD'S MUSHROOM)
AGARICUS BLAZEI

HISTORY

This mushroom's first appearance occurs in medical treatises from the Byzantine Empire. It also shows up in the Amazon rainforest, valued by the people of this region for bringing longevity and health. Considered more than just a food there, its name reveals its importance: "the mushroom of God."

In the 1960s, Takatoshi Furumoto became seriously interested in this mushroom. Since then, researchers have delved into its many health benefits.[1] In the Piedade region, where the mushroom is grown and consumed, the inhabitants' unusually low rate of geriatric illness has caught the attention of researchers, leading the mushroom's popularity to skyrocket. Its cultivation is now being attempted worldwide.

- Cancer fighter
- Immunity booster
- Diabetic aid
- Counteracts chemo-
  therapy side effects
- Osteoporosis preventer

DOSAGE

Depending on intended use, the dosage will differ.

For diabetes control: extract 500 mg, up to three times a day.

BENEFITS

Himematsutake is still being researched, but it is proving one of the most hopeful anticancer solutions to date, with a well-organized, broad spectrum of immune-support factors. It can also be used to improve the body's insulin intake and decrease insulin resistance in people with Type II diabetes. Those seeking to lower their cholesterol, improve digestive problems, and reduce the side-effects of chemotherapy should consider God's mushroom.[2] It can also be effective in preventing heart disease, osteoporosis, and stomach ulcers.

SAFETY

The mushroom has been shown to lower blood sugar. Do not use it while pregnant or breastfeeding. If you have liver disease, avoid adding it to your routine. Always consult a physician before adding himematsutake to your diet.

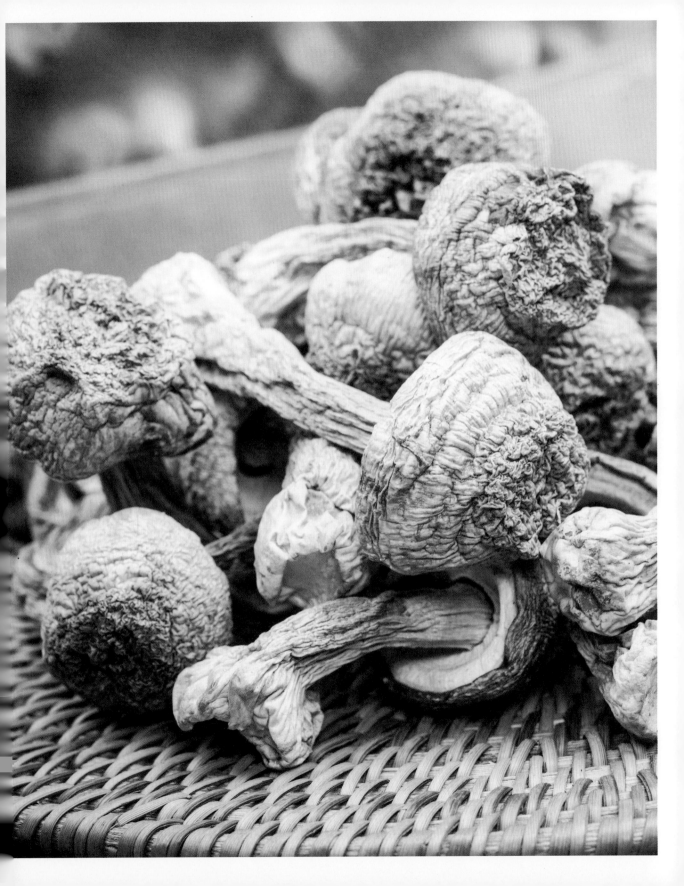

ALBIZIA

ALBIZIA JULIBRISSIN

HISTORY

This silk plant has a beautiful tasseled flower and is easily identifiable by its leaf shape. The bark and flower are both used in TCM. It is said that the bark has a more calming effect and the flowers have a more elevating one. In general, this plant is used to combat anxiety and stress.

- Sleep problems
- Anxiety/depression
- Sore throat
- Antidiarrheal

DOSAGE

The most common form of this adaptogen is as an extract.

Take 30 to 60 drops, up to three times a day.

BENEFITS

Incredibly helpful in treating diarrhea, insomnia, and poor memory. Albizia bark is also highly prized as an herbal supplement when recovering from physical trauma. It functions as an analgesic, nerve relaxant, and sedative.

SAFETY

Do *not* use albizia while pregnant. Can also have adverse effects to anesthesia. Do not take at least two weeks prior to scheduled surgery. Always consult your physician before adding it to your routine.

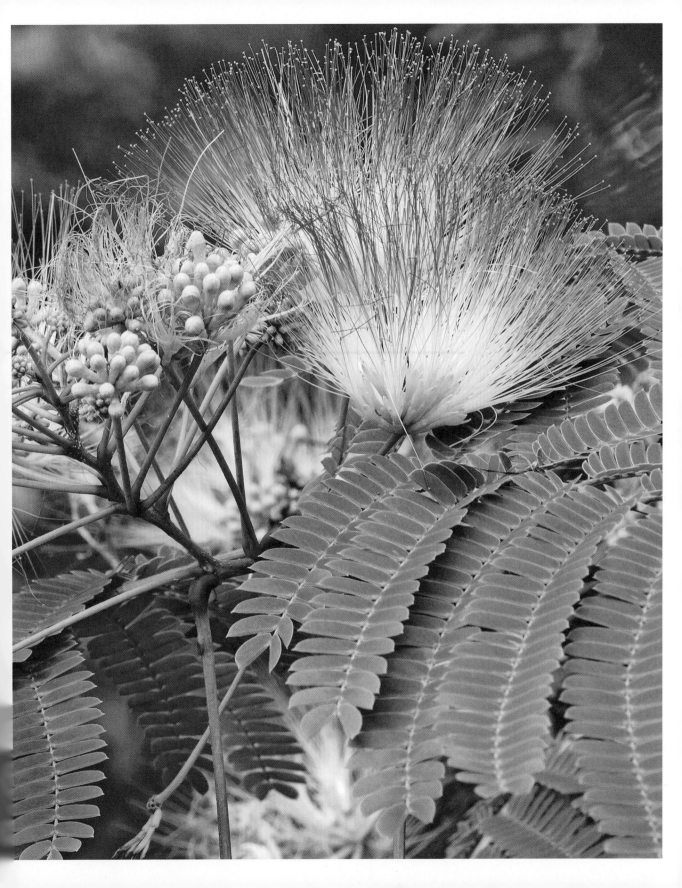

ASHITABA
ANGELICA KEISKEI

HISTORY

Ashitaba is native to Japan, primarily its central region. The root, leaf, and stem are used in making medicine. In Japan it is celebrated as a beauty food that offers anti-aging benefits. The leaves and roots appear in regional cuisine such as soba, tempura, ice cream, and sochu. It has also been recognized as a major contributor to the healthier, extended lives enjoyed by the people of this part of Japan. Ashitaba was used to treat smallpox and currently serves as a diuretic, digestion aid, and, when applied topically, promotes healing and resistance to infection.

- Concentration and focus
- Digestive aid
- Increased milk supply
- Vitamins B6 and B12 for vegans
- Longevity

DOSAGE

Take 2.68 g in 20:1 concentrated extract. Other concentrates may differ.

BENEFITS

Ashitaba has been shown to help with concentration and focus, wound healing, infection resistance, and healthy digestion. As a source for vitamins B6 and B12, it's especially beneficial for vegans. It has also been shown to encourage nerve growth hormones, which could explain its reputation for increasing longevity. Another of its powers is a reported ability to increase milk supply in breastfeeding mothers.

SAFETY

Always consult your physician before adding it to your routine.

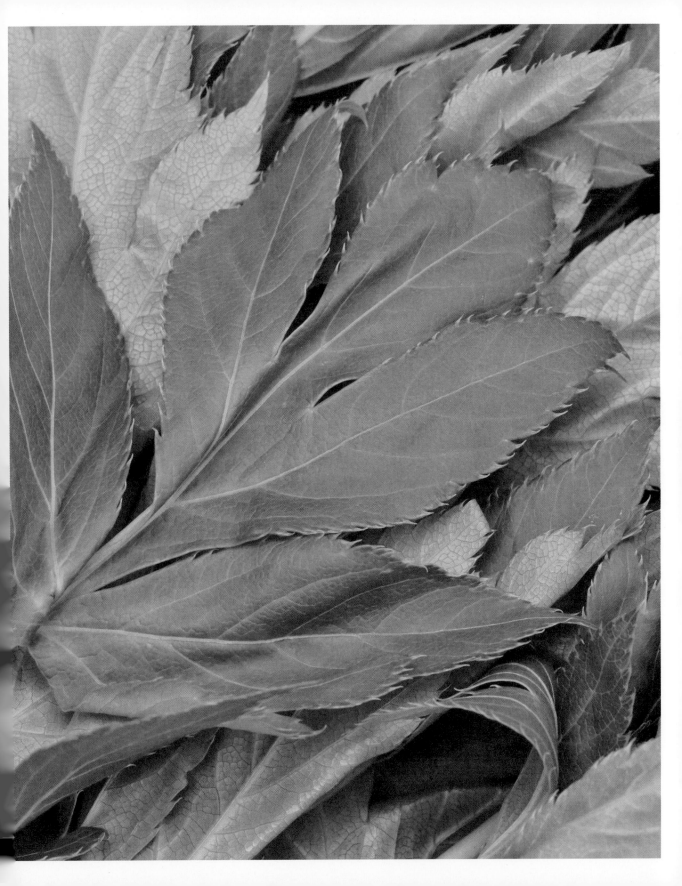

BURDOCK
ARTICIUM LAPPA

HISTORY

Burdock root is native to northern Asia and Europe. It was traditionally used in Chinese medicine as a digestive aid and diuretic. It has been given many names over time, including beggar's buttons, bardana, clothburr, cockle buttons, fox's clote, Gypsy rhubarb, and thorny burr. In Japan, they call it *gobo* and use it in many savory dishes. It has been used as a vegetable in soups and stews in the United States, and has become a popular addition to salads since the 1980s.

Most of burdock's medicinal benefits are stored in its roots, which are long, dark black, and gangly looking. The roots contain alkaloids, inulin, essential oils, flavonoids, resin, tannins, and volatile oil. The seeds are a good source of vitamins A and B and essential fatty acids. The seeds and leaves have been found to have a soothing quality to the mucous membranes in the body. In most historical references, burdock is used as a blood purifier, promoter of perspiration, and purgative of toxins from the body.

- Digestion
- Liver health
- Treatment of psoriasis and eczema
- Restores gut health after antibiotics

DOSAGE

Varies greatly, depending on the issue being treated.

BENEFITS

This herb has so many benefits, it's hard to focus on just a few. Historically, it was used primarily as a blood purifier. It stimulates the secretion of bile, making it a good digestive herb while also aiding liver function. It has also been shown to clear up psoriasis and eczema and to restore intestinal flora in the body after antibiotic use; it may also bring some relief for chronic arthritis and gout. Mild and lightly sweet, burdock root can be peeled and added to soups, salads, and stews.

SAFETY

This root is not recommended for pregnant or breastfeeding women. You should also consult your physician if you are diabetic and wish to add it to your diet: some cases show that burdock interacts with medications given to control diabetes. Always consult your physician before adding it to your routine.

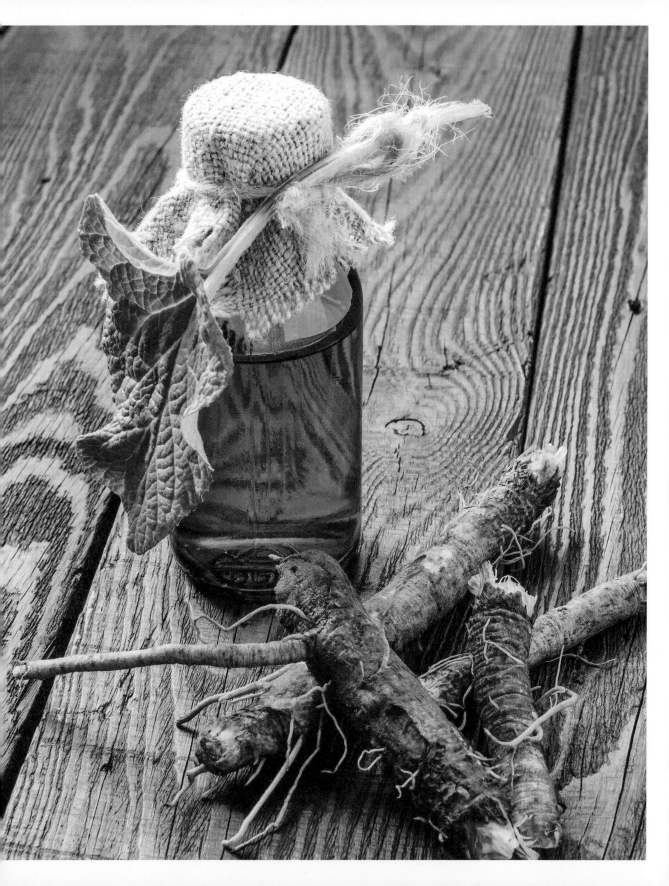

SHATAVARI
ASPARAGUS RACEMOSUS

HISTORY

Shatavari has a long association with Ayurveda. Its name has two meanings: "She who has hundreds of husbands" and "one hundred roots." Both names are fitting indeed, since Ayurveda identifies this type of wild asparagus as essential for women's health and fertility. It has a slender, aboveground stalk, but its underground section possesses hundreds of thick, succulent roots. The plant was traditionally used for bladder inflammation and to rid the body of sticky mucous accompanying a persistent cough.

- Aphrodisiac
- Female reproductive health
- Gut health
- Immune system support
- Fatigue fighter
- Hormone harmonizer

BENEFITS

This herb is high in saponins, compounds with antioxidant properties; these help prevent cell damage from free radicals. Shatavari also offers impressive anti-inflammatory properties without causing distress to the digestive system. While there are many other benefits offered by this plant—including treating diarrhea, acting as a diuretic, helping relieve coughs, strengthening the immune system, working to heal ulcers, and reducing kidney stones—shatavari's main benefit is in supporting women's health. Easing menopause symptoms, stimulating the libido, resetting minor hormone imbalances, and boosting fertility are all benefits of this powerful adaptogen. Breastfeeding women may even find that this plant helps increase their milk flow.

DOSAGE

Take 40 to 80 drops of extract up to three times a day, or take the dried herb 1 to 2 teaspoons, up to two times a day.

SAFETY

Shatavari is a mild diuretic, so if you are on any diuretics or prescription medications that are excreted through the kidneys, this may not be for you. It is also not indicated for those with a history of estrogen receptor-positive cancer. Always consult with your physician before adding shatavari to your routine.

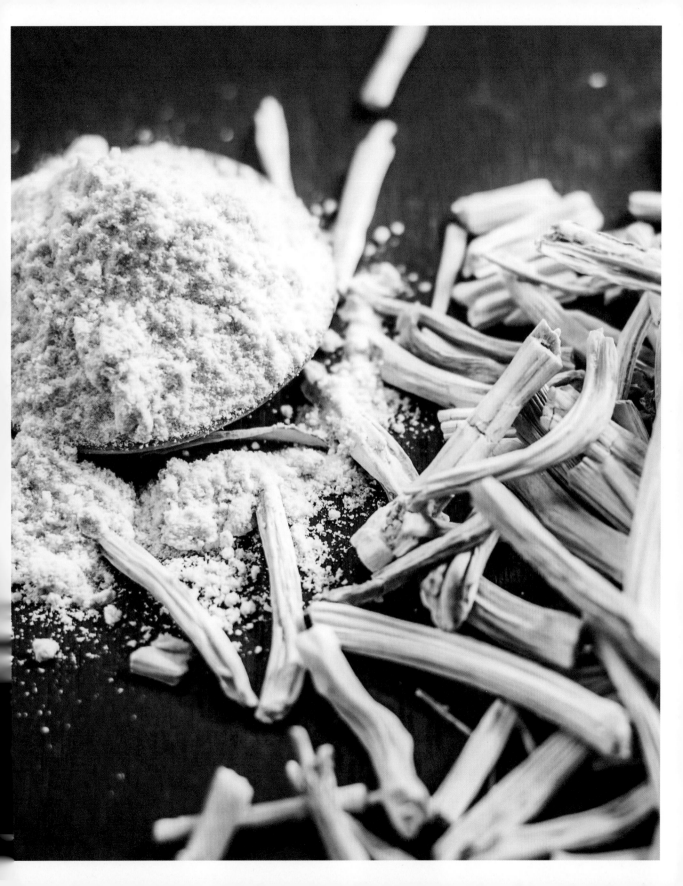

ASTRAGALUS
ASTRAGALUS MEMBRANACEUS

HISTORY

This mild plant root has long been used in Traditional Chinese Medicine. It originally grew wild in China, Mongolia, Korea, and Siberia, but today it is mainly cultivated. This tonic has been used in TCM for centuries to protect the body from disease and to support the liver.

• Immunity booster

• Speedy flu recovery

• Whole body

DOSAGE

Take 40 to 80 drops of extract up to three times a day.

BENEFITS

Astragalus is known for having many health benefits; its immune-boosting, anti-aging, and anti-inflammatory effects being just a few. It is said that astragalus can extend one's life. Its less famous benefits include treating fatigue, allergies, and even the common cold. The beauty of this adaptogen lies in the fact that it is beneficial for the immune, cardiovascular, nervous, and digestive systems, making it beneficial for the entire body. Whether this intelligent plant is ingested to recover from a specific illness or taken regularly, it is a great support for complete health.

SAFETY

Astragalus is traditionally not taken during acute illness, so avoid it while you're still contagious. It is said that it prolongs fever. It may also alter other medications, so always check with your physician before adding it into your routine. It should also be avoided during pregnancy and breastfeeding. It has been shown to be safe for use with children.

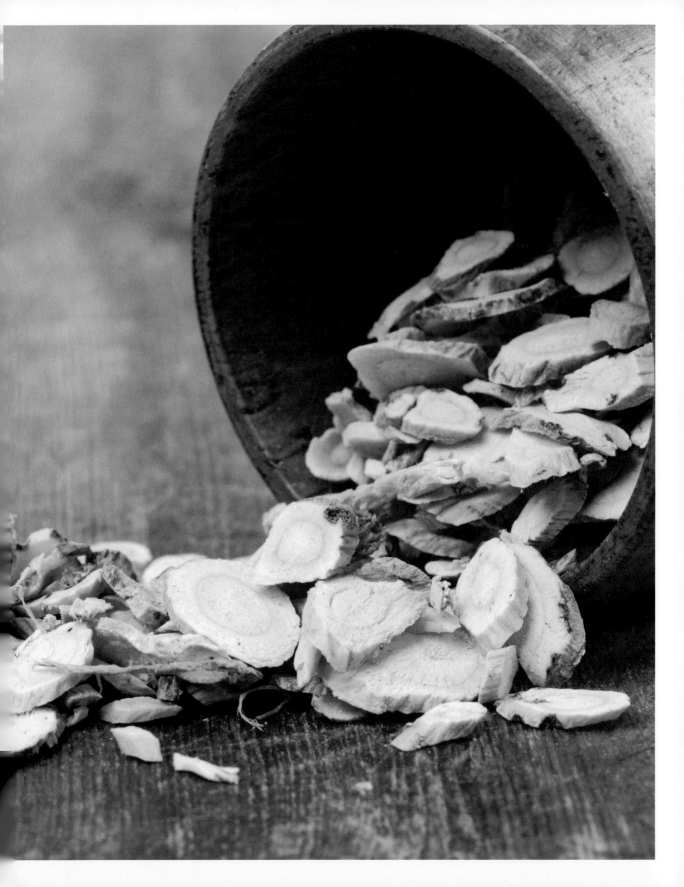

BACOPA
BACOPA MONNIERI

HISTORY

This adaptogen is also known as brahmi, water hyssop, thyme-leaved gratiola, and herb of grace. It has long been used in traditional Ayurvedic medicine to increase certain brain chemicals that are involved in memory, learning, and thinking.

- Improve memory and protect brain cells
- Concentration
- Inflammation fighter
- ADHD symptoms
- Stress and anxiety helper

DOSAGE

Can range from 300 to 450 mg per day.

BENEFITS

This plant has been beneficial in the treatment of Alzheimer's disease because of its capacity to improve memory and protect brain cells.[3] It has also been shown to aid in the treatment of anxiety and attention deficit hyperactivity disorder (ADHD). Treating epilepsy is also one of its many powers. Including this plant in your routine has also been shown to reduce anxiety. Bacopa interacts with the dopamine and serotonergic systems, but its primary action is to promote neuron communication by increasing the growth of nerve endings. It is also an antioxidant that has been shown to prevent the damage caused by free radicals. Lowering blood pressure, reducing inflammation, and containing anticancer properties are a few of its other superpowers.

SAFETY

Bacopa is not safe for pregnant and breastfeeding women. It has also been shown to slow heart rates, so those with a heart condition should avoid it. Some studies have shown that bacopa might increase secretions in the stomach and intestines. Avoid this one if you have ulcers. It's best to take it on a full stomach; taking it on an empty stomach can cause bloating, cramps, nausea, and diarrhea. Always consult with your physician before adding bacopa to your routine.

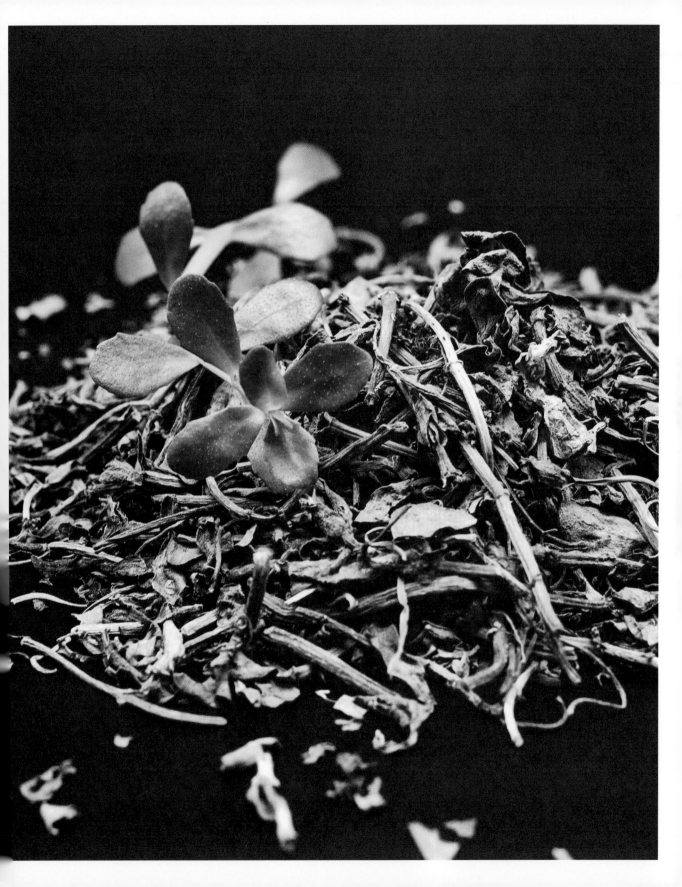

GOTU KOLA
CENTELLA ASIATICA

HISTORY

This powerful herb is known as the "herb of longevity." Gotu kola has been used in Ayurvedic and Chinese medicine as an immune system equalizer, helping boost mental clarity, heal skin issues, serve as a nervous system and thyroid tonic, and promote cardiovascular health. Some consider this herb to be a nootropic, that is, an herb that can improve cognitive functions, especially memory, creativity, and motivation.

- Heart health
- Immune support
- Thyroid stimulant
- Harmonizer
- Cognitive health
- Autoimmune disorders
- Stress and anxiety buster
- Detoxifier

DOSAGE

Take 40 to 60 drops of extract up to three times a day, or take the dried herb, 1 to 2 teaspoons, up to three times a day.

BENEFITS

One of the most wonderful things about this intelligent plant is that it combines its immune-harmonizing properties with its vulnerary ones. A vulnerary herb is one that aids in the healing of the skin and tissues, whether internal or external. Gotu kola's anti-inflammatory properties, in combination with its immune-harmonizing and vulnerary ones, make this herb great for fighting autoimmune diseases such as allergy-related skin disorders, inflammatory disorders within the digestive tract, and rheumatoid arthritis. This adaptogen is also effective in supporting mental clarity and focus. There have even been a few studies showing that it is linked with improving mental and neural health in Alzheimer's disease patients.[4] Other studies have found that gotu kola may help lessen anxiety and stress, act as an antidepressant, improve circulation and swelling, help sufferers of insomnia, lessen the presence of stretch marks, reduce scarring, advance wound healing, relieve joint pain, and have a natural detoxifying effect.

SAFETY

This herb is best used when starting with a small amount and gradually increasing as needed. It has been shown to cause headaches, stomach upset, and dizziness. Gotu kola is one of those adaptogens that is best taken sporadically. Two to six weeks on and then two weeks off is recommended. You should not take it if you are pregnant or breastfeeding or have any disease of the liver. Always consult with your physician before adding gotu kola to your routine.

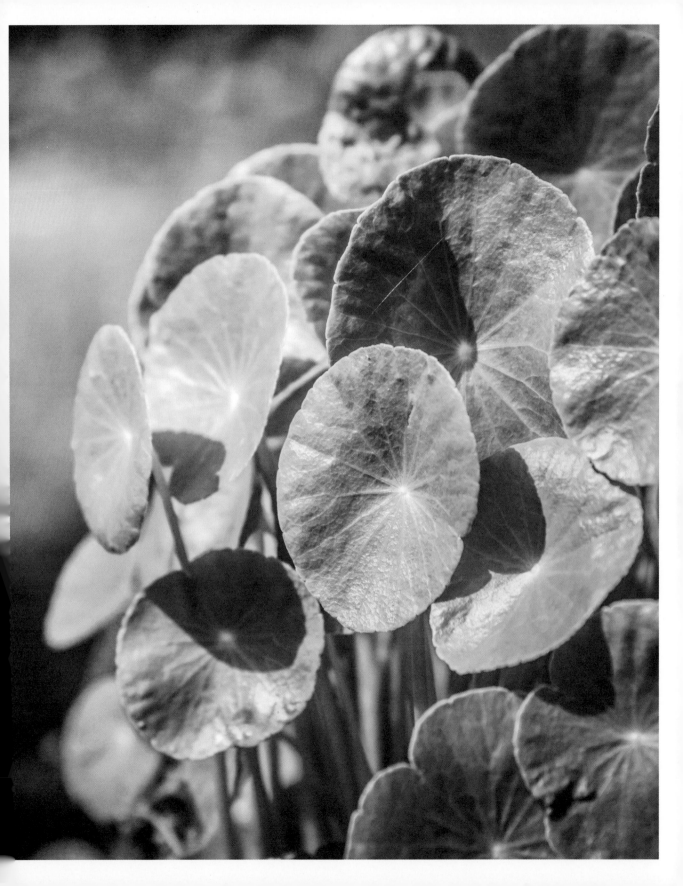

DANG SHEN
CODONOPSIS PILOSULA

HISTORY

Use of this beautiful flowering vine was first recorded in China in 1670. It was often used as a less expensive alternative to ginseng. Although it is milder than ginseng, it has a great reputation for improving digestion, building the blood, and supporting the immune system. It is a mild adaptogen that is widely used in Traditional Chinese Medicine as a superb and potent qi tonic. In China, it has been widely used for building strong muscles in children.

- Immunity support
- Spleen and lung health
- Fatigue fighter
- Elderly immune booster

DOSAGE

Take 40 to 80 drops of extract up to three times a day, or 1 to 2 teaspoons of dried root in 8 ounces of hot water, two times a day.

BENEFITS

Dang shen is effective for invigorating the spleen and lungs. It has also been shown to relieve a general sense of fatigue, making it really useful for women during their menstrual cycle because it also helps build blood. It has a very powerful way of strengthening the digestive, respiratory, and immune systems. It's rich in polysaccharides as well, making it highly beneficial for supporting the immune systems of the elderly.

SAFETY

Dang shen is not suitable for those with high iron levels, as it has been shown to increase hemoglobin counts. It is also not traditionally used to treat acute illness such as cold and flu. Always consult your physician before adding it to your routine.

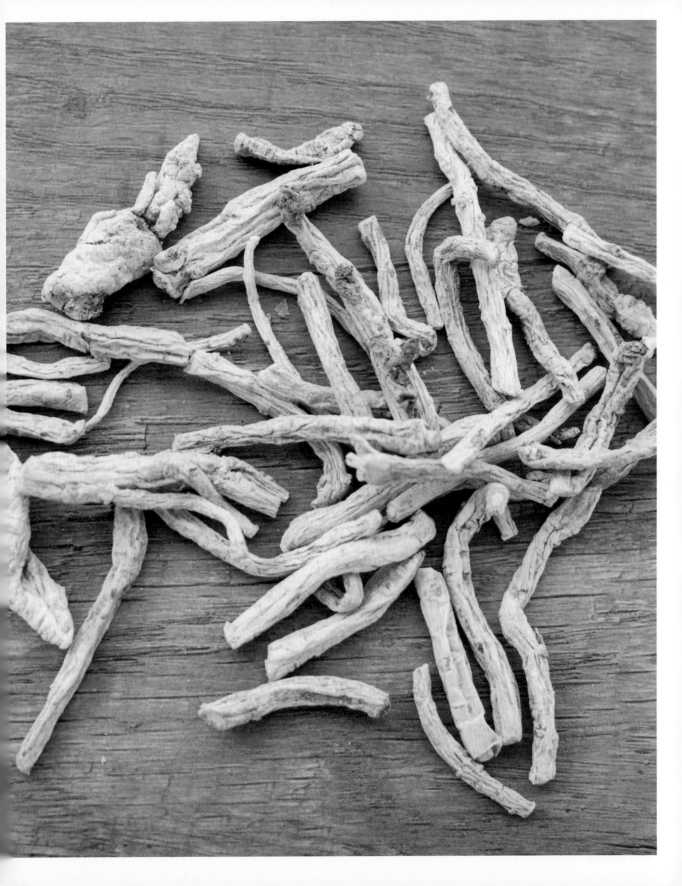

CORDYCEPS
CORDYCEPS SINENSIS

HISTORY

This fungus has quite an interesting origin. The cordyceps mushroom is a type of fungus that lives within caterpillars. The fungus consumes the larvae of the ghost moth, then it surrounds the caterpillar and produces a mushroom to release its spores. For practical storage, the mushroom and caterpillar are dried. These mushrooms have always been coveted, because they are so rare. In the 1700s, Traditional Chinese Medicine only served their medicinal magic to nobility and emperors, but these days we have found a way to produce and cultivate them using soy instead of caterpillars, bringing their medicinal properties to the masses. They were traditionally used to support the health of the kidneys and defend against infertility, sexual dysfunction, frequent urination, night sweats, ringing in the ears, and fatigue.

- Immunity support
- Energy booster
- Fertility
- Liver and kidney support
- Endurance

DOSAGE

Take in extract form, 20 to 40 drops up to three times a day, or 1 to 2 cups of tea made from ¼ to ½ teaspoon of dried cordyceps.

BENEFITS

Today we use cordyceps for all its incredible medicinal benefits. It is widely known to support the hormonal, or endocrine system, and to create a sense of homeostasis during stressful times. This mushroom has been shown to support mental and physical endurance as well as the immune system. Some studies show that this mushroom enhances physical performance by increasing the body's production of ATP, which is vital for carrying oxygen to your body and delivering energy to muscles. As in the past, this fungus is still used as an aphrodisiac and supposedly improves overall sexual vigor.

SAFETY

Consuming too many of these mushrooms can be a bad thing. Anxiety, weakened immune system, and water retention have all been experienced when too much of this mushroom is ingested. There are also some studies that show that they interact with immunosuppressive medications. Always consult your physician before adding it to your routine.

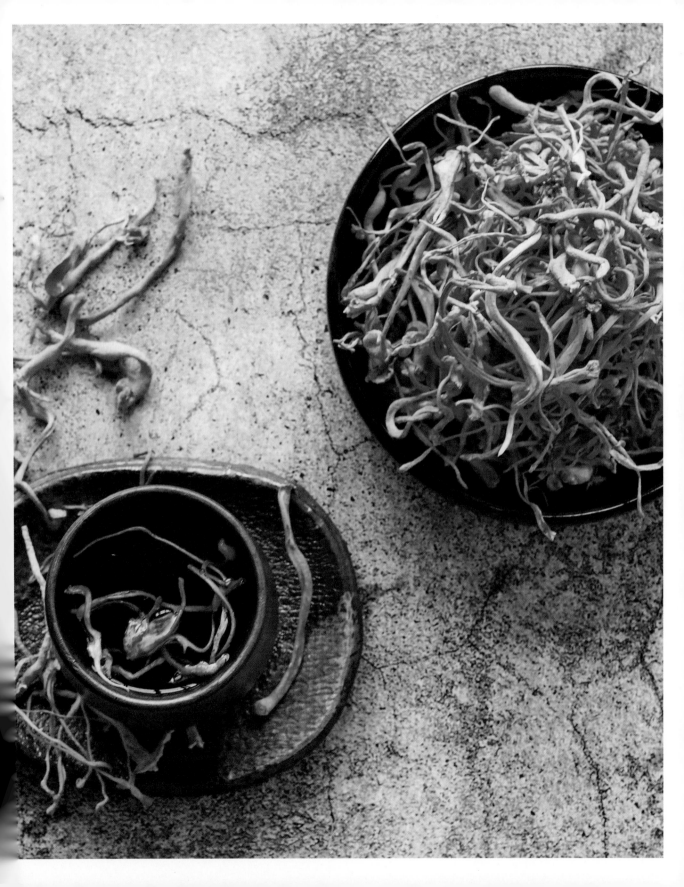

ELEUTHERO
(SIBERIAN GINSENG)
ELEUTHEROCOCCUS SENTICOSUS

HISTORY

This was the first plant to be classified as an adaptogen. Even though it is not in the same class of plants as other ginsengs, it is sometimes called Siberian ginseng because of the similarities to other ginsengs. It is native to Siberia, China, Korea, and Japan. It is much milder than the *panax* form of ginseng and has long since been used in China as a medicinal wine to help recover from low energy.

- Immune support
- Endurance
- Alertness
- Muscle building

DOSAGE

Typically, 50 to 100 drops of the extract are taken up to three times a day, or the dried herb, ½ to 1 teaspoon, can be taken once a day.

BENEFITS

This well-rounded plant can be used by men and women, as well as the elderly. Its super-gentle, supportive nature makes it great for long-term use. In Traditional Chinese Medicine, eleuthero has been used in many different ways, everything from offering cognitive support and supporting the immune system to invigorating sexual function and maintaining healthy cholesterol levels. It's considered beneficial to heart health and to supporting endurance in athletes by shortening recovery time. This mild adaptogen is a great one to include in one's diet for optimal health.

SAFETY

Eleuthero is often said to work best when you take it in bursts. Try one month on, two months off for best results. It is also counterindicated for those on some medicines, especially heart medications. Always consult with your physician before adding it to your routine.

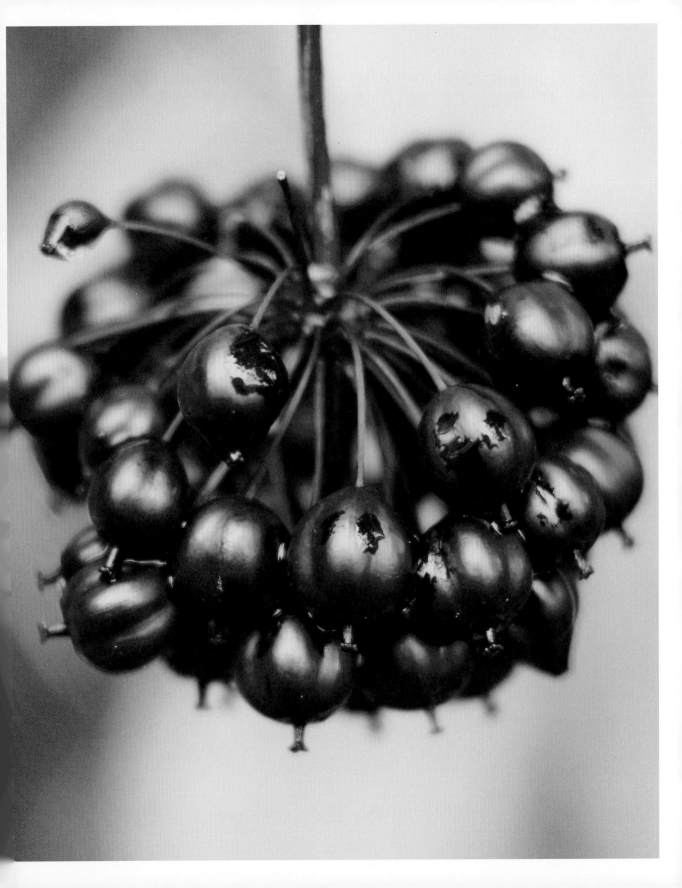

AMLA (INDIAN GOOSEBERRY)
EMBLICA OFFICINALIS
(SYN. PHYLLANTHUS EMBLICA)

HISTORY

This intelligent plant has deep Ayurvedic roots. It's commonly known as Indian gooseberry or amalaki. It is native to southern China, India, Sri Lanka, Myanmar, and Malaysia.

• Immune booster
• Seasonal depression
• Glowing skin
• Regularity

DOSAGE

Take ½ to 1 teaspoon of amla fruit in a beverage, or 60 to 90 drops of 1:4 or 1:5 extract. It may be taken up to three times a day.

BENEFITS

In Ayurveda, amla is one of those plants that is known as a rasayana. It is believed to prolong life, good memory, and youthfulness. It serves as the common base for an Ayurvedic blend called *chyawanprash*, which is a highly potent blend of herbs, spices, and adaptogens.

More than merely an adaptogen, amla is rich in vitamin C and antioxidants. Its benefits include, but are not limited to: increasing resistance to disease, nourishing the blood, restoring the appetite, supporting liver health, and supporting the health of bones, teeth, and hair. Its capacity to balance the delicate intestinal mucous lends itself to benefiting not only the gut but the skin as well. It is also a light laxative, which is why it is used in Ayurvedic blends to help support proper elimination.

SAFETY

Taking amla might interfere with iron absorption because of the tannins it contains. Staggering ingestion of this herb between doses of other medications can help increase their effectiveness, especially alkaloid ones. Always consult your physician before adding it to your routine.

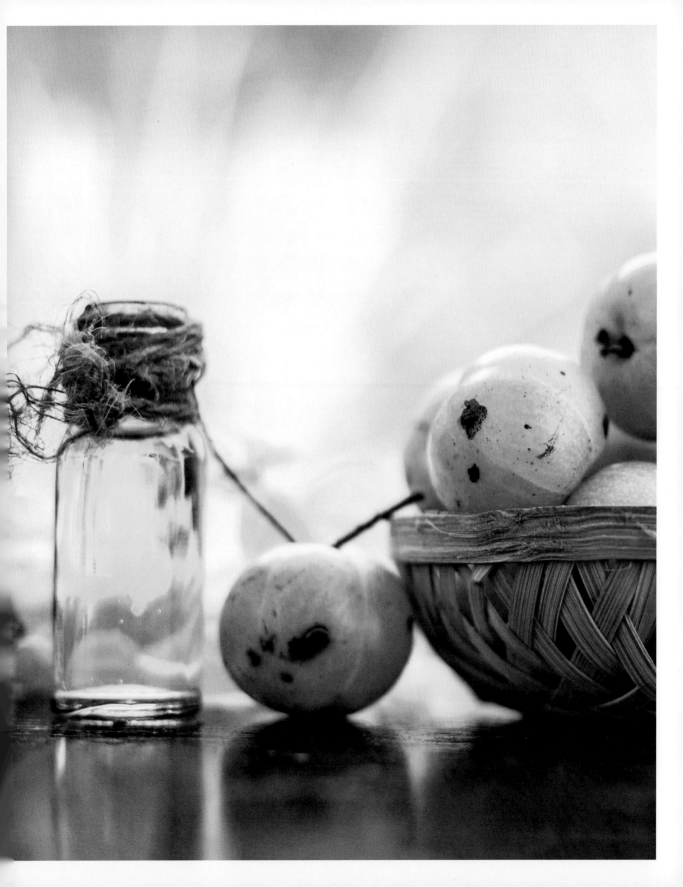

REISHI
GANODERMA LUCIDUM

HISTORY

This mushroom dates back over two thousand years to the Han dynasty, where it was known as the "elixir of immortality." In ancient texts, the Reishi mushroom is described as having therapeutic properties, tonifying effects, a strengthening cardiac function, and the ability to enhance qi. It can be used for increasing memory functions and enhancing anti-aging effects. Originally available only to Chinese nobles, the mushroom's notoriety has grown so vast that it is now the most researched plant in the world.

- Antiviral
- Heart health
- Immune support
- Anxiety and depression
- Sleep helper
- Seasonal allergies

DOSAGE

Take 80 to 100 drops of extract, up to six times a day.

BENEFITS

There are few areas in the body that this mushroom doesn't support.

Let's look at its immune-boosting properties. Reishi contains beta-D glucan, which aids in boosting and enhancing the immune system while also reducing swelling with its anti-inflammatory properties. This mushroom basically teaches your immune system, even as it ages, to work smarter, not harder.

Reishi's reign comes into play with its major stress-relieving powers. It aids the physiological response to stress by calming the mind and relaxing the body. The reishi mushroom has also received a lot of attention for its ability to curb severe high blood pressure, with results that indicate it can indeed be beneficial in lowering high blood pressure. It has also been studied for its ability to increase good HDL cholesterol and to lower triglycerides.

Reishi is also a histamine regulator, which means if you suffer from pet, pollen, or seasonal allergies, this adaptogen will help regulate the amount of histamines released by the body when you come into contact with said allergen. A few of its more potent benefits include promoting longevity, reducing insomnia, providing massive antioxidants, and serving as an anti-inflammatory.

SAFETY

Avoid the reishi if you're allergic to other mushrooms. It should also be avoided if you are on blood-thinning medications. Always consult with your physician before adding it to your routine.

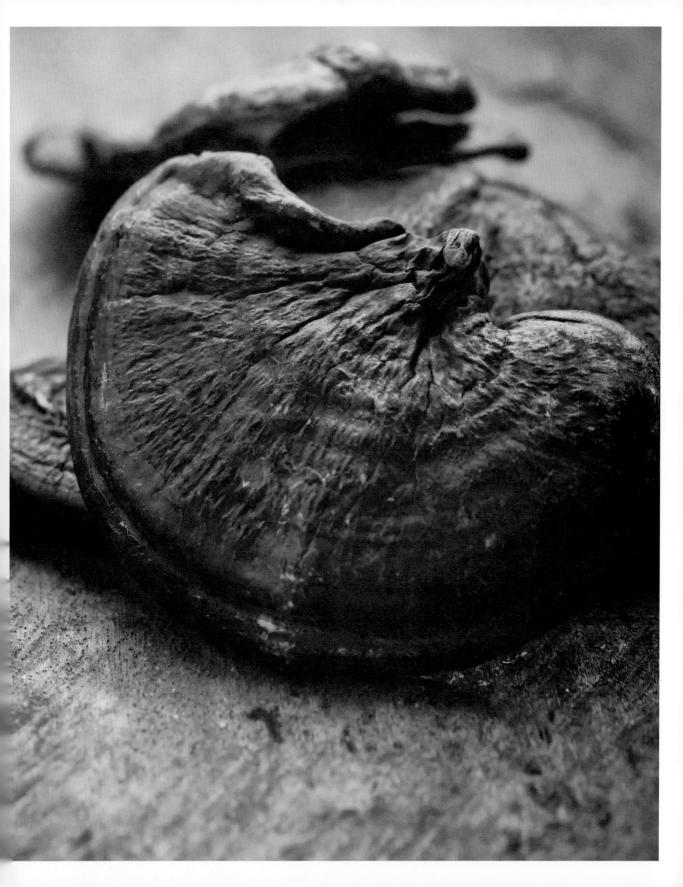

LION'S MANE
HERICIUM ERINACEUS

HISTORY

This super-mushroom, also known as the hedgehog mushroom, has long been used in Traditional Chinese Medicine for its brain and neurological health benefits, as well as offering stress support. While not widely used, it was rather reserved for royalty as both a medicine and culinary treat. Traditionally, TCM employed the mushroom as a preventative for gastrointestinal cancer. Nevertheless, it is not clear if this mushroom is classified as an adaptogen yet, but it does meet all criteria.

• Concentration

• Brain booster

• Anxiety and depression

• Immune support

• Heart health

• Wound healing

DOSAGE

Differs depending on function.

BENEFITS

The lion's mane mushroom's properties are phenomenal, including antibacterial, anticandida, antitumor, and anti-inflammatory benefits. It can also be used in a nerve tonic.

Recent studies have focused on this mushroom's capability to stimulate the growth of neurons in the brain. It has been shown to help with Alzheimer's, Parkinson's, and multiple sclerosis. The lion's mane contains nerve growth factors, which aid in the regeneration and protection of brain tissue. Some other superlative benefits include lowering depression and anxiety, aiding in heart health, creating a healthy immune response, and aiding in wound healing.

SAFETY

Always consult your physician before adding this mushroom to your routine.

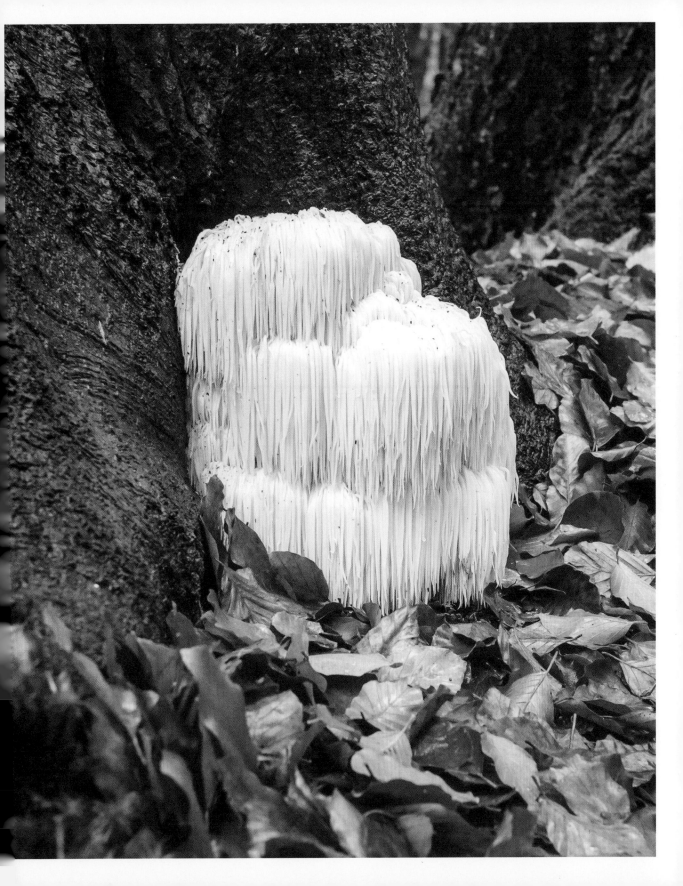

SEA BUCKTHORN

HIPPOPHAE

HISTORY

Sea buckthorn is a powerhouse that has thrived in the harsh conditions and high altitude of the Himalayas. It was first documented around thirteen centuries ago in the Tibetan book of healing arts called *Sibu Yi Dian*; over a third of the pages are devoted to this incredible fruit and its many uses. This berry has unparalleled levels of omega-3, -6, and -9, and even contains the obscure omega-7, which is an essential fatty acid that is fundamental for collagen production and for healthy skin, hair, and nails. Genghis Khan used sea buckthorn to power his army and horses. It was used to fortify Greek horses and was said to keep their coats shiny. This berry was also used to help protect the skin from the harmful effects of the sun and other elements.

- Skin health
- Eczema and rosacea symptoms
- Healthy inflammation response
- Decreases wrinkles
- Heart health
- Joint support
- Collagen production
- Gut health
- Weight loss
- Longevity

DOSAGE

The right dose depends on factors, including your reasons for taking it.

BENEFITS

This versatile little orange berry is said to aid in the treatment of the common cold and the flu, thanks to being an incredible antioxidant and immunity support. The omegas in the berry are responsible for collagen production, improved cellular health, moisturizing dry and damaged skin, decreasing fine lines and wrinkles, treating skin ailments such as psoriasis, eczema, and rosacea, and helping overall nourishment of the skin. This adaptogen is also remarkable for aiding in gut health and digestion, strengthening the immune system, lubricating joints, aiding in arthritic pain, and helping support weight loss.

SAFETY

Sea buckthorn has been shown to slow blood clotting. Always consult your physician before adding it to your routine.

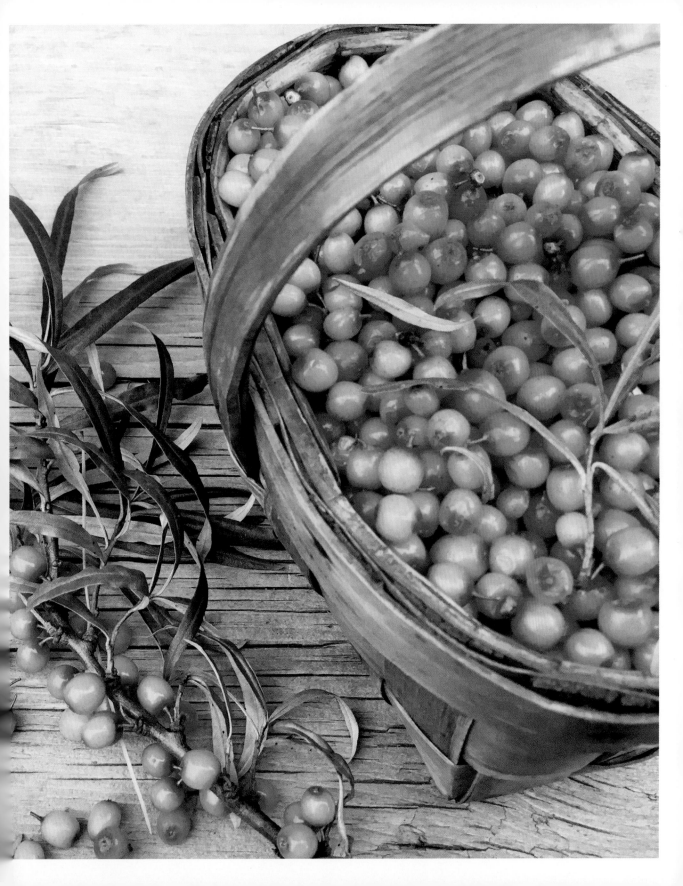

SHIITAKE
HONGOS SHIITAKE

HISTORY

The shiitake mushroom in Traditional Chinese Medicine is depicted in tapestries woven over five thousand years ago. These medicinal mushrooms were used as aphrodisiacs and promoters of youthfulness and virility.

- Youthfulness
- Virility
- Aphrodisiac
- Immune booster

DOSAGE

The dosage of shiitake mushroom extract differs greatly from one application to the next.

BENEFITS

Today the shiitake mushroom is beloved in all its culinary aspects, but its medicinal benefits still take the main stage. An extract made from this mushroom works as an incredible immune booster. Its powers are so strong, in fact, that it is often used in conjunction with HIV/AIDS medications to boost immunity.[5] This mushroom is also known to lower blood cholesterol levels, aid in diabetic control, treat eczema, reduce cold and flu symptoms, and support recovery from prostate and breast cancer; it is used in many anti-aging tonics. New ways to use this extract include the treatment of hepatitis B, herpes, and high blood pressure.

SAFETY

While whole shiitake mushrooms are safe for consumption, the shiitake mushroom extract is not safe for those who are pregnant or breastfeeding. The extract may also cause the immune system to become more active; for this reason, those with autoimmune diseases should avoid this adaptogen. Always consult with your physician before adding this extract to your routine.

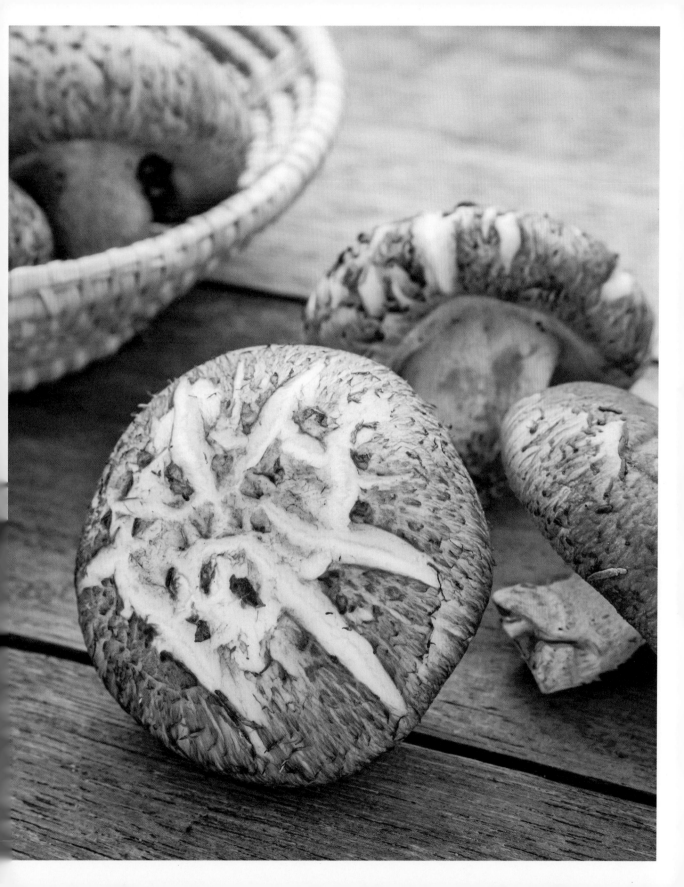

CHAGA
INONOTUS OBLIQUUS

HISTORY

This mushroom, originally found in the birch forests of Russia and northern Europe, is a parasite that grows from the inside of the birch tree outward. The mushroom is known by several names, including black mass, clinker polypore, birch canker polypore, cinder conk, and the sterile conk trunk rot. In Russia and other northern European countries, it has been used to boost immunity and enhance overall health. Its burnt charcoal mass was typically dried, ground, and brewed into teas.

- Immunity support
- Anxiety
- Anticarcinogen
- Travel support

DOSAGE

Take up to 3.5 g daily.

BENEFITS

Strengthening and supporting the immune system are the main properties of this mushroom. Rich in beta-D glucans, which have been shown to support healthy immune functions, this adaptogen offers the capacity to speed up a lethargic immune system or slow down an overcharged one. Chaga is also great for fighting long-term inflammation and harmful bacteria and viruses. Its use as a stimulant is well attested, thanks to the nutrients and antioxidants it contains that can pick you up without making you jittery like traditional caffeine. Chaga makes an excellent travel companion for this reason. It's considered anticarcinogenic because of its high antioxidant content, which protects the body from free radicals.

SAFETY

Chaga may interfere with certain prescribed medications. Always consult your physician before adding it to your routine. Some studies have shown that it contains a protein that can hinder blood clotting.

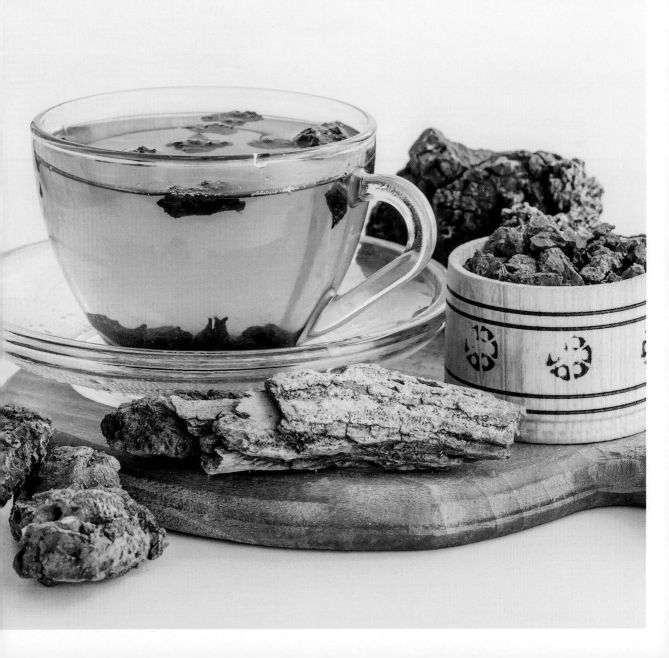

MACA

LEPIDIUM MEYENII

HISTORY

Maca is considered one of the "lost crops of the Andes." It grows in the extreme conditions of the Andes mountains of South America, which makes it rare, though it is also one of the area's primary food sources. There is some record of Incan soldiers carrying the root with them into battle to enhance their endurance, strength, and fierceness. Maca was traditionally reserved for the royal court and imperial family, used as currency for trade as well as a powerful medicine.

- Aphrodisiac
- Sperm count booster
- Mood enhancer
- Menopause symptoms
- Immune booster
- Nutrition powerhouse

DOSAGE

Take in dried form up to 1,000 to 1,500 mg per day, two times a day.

BENEFITS

This nutritious root has a reputation for being an aphrodisiac and a hormone balancer, beneficial for improving menopausal symptoms, increasing male and female fertility, helping to correct erectile dysfunction, and boosting both male and female libido. Maca is also a great mood enhancer for when you're a little down. Its nutritional content is not to be ignored, either: maca offers substantial amounts of potassium, magnesium, calcium, iron, and iodine. This root is also a great source of vitamin C, making it a great immune booster.

SAFETY

This cruciferous vegetable contains high levels of glucosinolates, which can have adverse effects on the thyroid. If you have thyroid problems, it is best to avoid this adaptogen. Always consult your physician before adding maca to your routine.

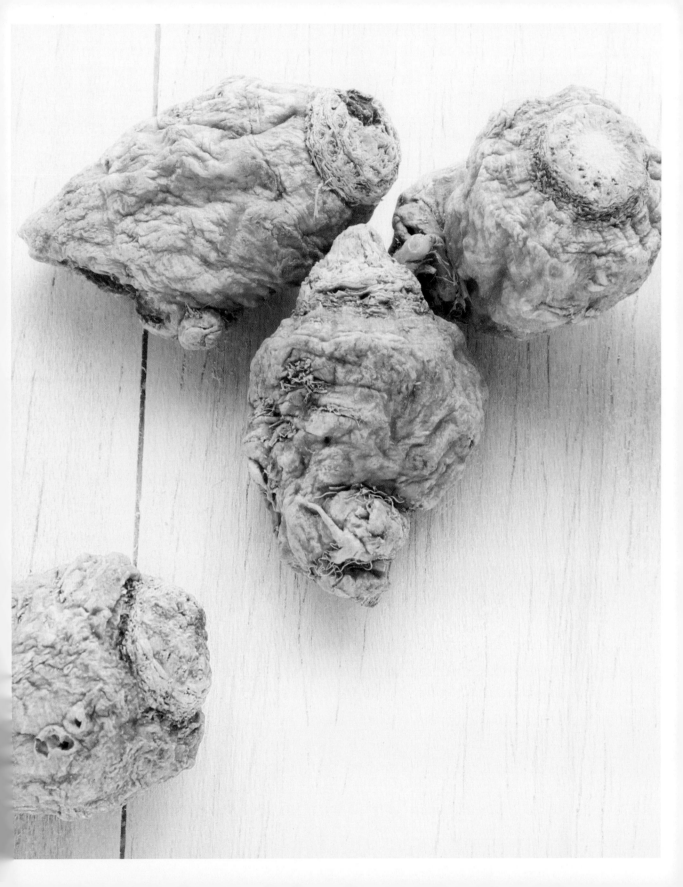

GOJI

LYCIUM BARBARUM

HISTORY

This superberry, also known as Chinese wolfberry, was traditionally used in Chinese medicine as a tonic to promote eye health. It is also used in combination with other herbs to promote the health of the liver, kidneys, and blood. The berry offers a phenomenal antioxidant load, which the body uses to fortify the veins, arteries, and capillaries.

- Immune support
- Longevity
- Anti-inflammatory
- Eye health

DOSAGE

Take 60 to 90 drops in extract form, three to four times a day. Or you can take one ounce of dried berries, or 1 to 2 teaspoons of dried and ground berries, one time a day.

BENEFITS

The goji berry contains all nine of the essential amino acids, and it's a great source of vitamin C. This berry is highly beneficial for eyesight, especially to support and assist with poor night vision, dry, red, or painful eyes, glaucoma, macular degeneration, and cataracts. It is also great for overall vitality.

SAFETY

The goji berry is part of the nightshade family. If you are sensitive to these plants, it is best to avoid this adaptogen. There are also some contraindications if you are taking the prescription medication warfarin, medications for diabetes, or some medications for blood pressure. Always consult your physician before adding it to your routine.

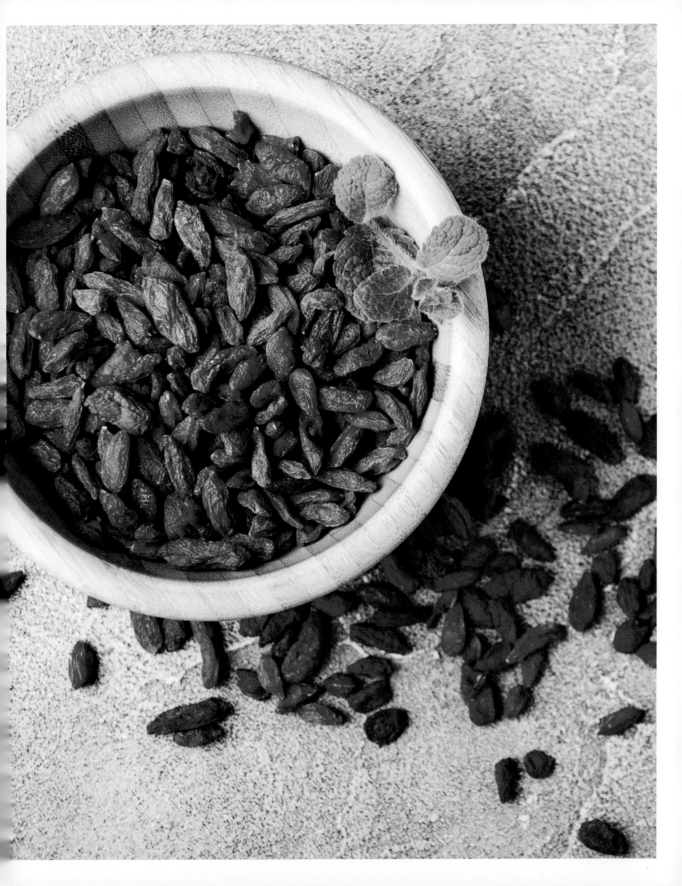

MORINGA
MORINGA OLEIFERA

HISTORY

This tree first shows up in history on the Indian subcontinent. Moringa was used in traditional Ayurvedic medicine to treat a wide variety of ailments, ranging from skin imperfections, asthma, blood pressure, kidney stones, and even tuberculosis. From India, news of its uses spread to ancient Egypt, Greece, and Rome. Its uses there ranged from a medicinal ointment to perfumes.

- Anxiety
- Digestion health
- Milk production
- Anti-aging
- Blood pressure lowering
- Skin health

DOSAGE

Dosage differs greatly, consult a physician.

BENEFITS

Moringa is a powerhouse of vitamins and minerals. It is an excellent source of vitamins A and E and antioxidants, making it highly beneficial for preventing skin damage and aiding in early signs of aging. It is also a great source of iron, vitamins B6, and C. This plant has been shown to lower cholesterol, reduce inflammation, aid in blood sugar control, balance hormones, and aid in digestion. Moringa contains tryptophan, an amino acid the body needs to create serotonin—which in turn helps stabilize one's mood. Another notable benefit of this tree is how fast it grows, even in dry, nutrient-depleted soil. Because of this, it is being used in reforestation and soil fertilization efforts.

SAFETY

Always buy from a reputable source. The root of the moringa may be toxic and should be avoided. Your package should state "moringa leaf powder." Always consult with a physician before adding it to your routine.

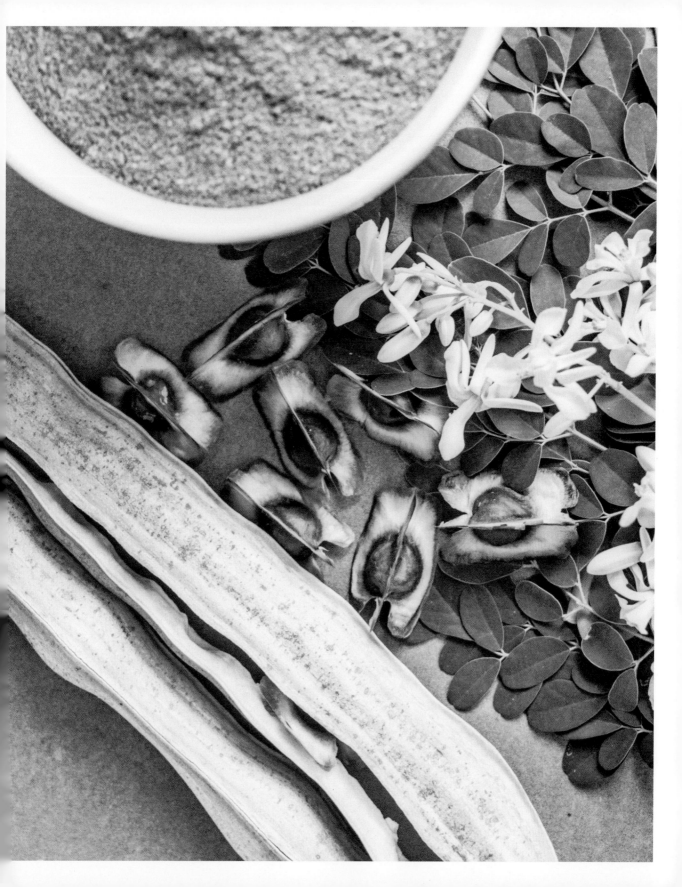

VELVET BEAN
MUCUNA PRURIENS

HISTORY

This leathery, hairy-podded bean has long been applied in Ayurvedic medicine as an aphrodisiac, useful for managing male infertility, nervous disorders, and, above all else, the treatment of Parkinson's disease. The antioxidant load of the velvet bean has been shown to have neuroprotective effects that counteract parkinsonism. Many indigenous cultures have used the beans as a source of nutrition and the beans' abundance of protein is said to have mood-lifting benefits. In Ayurveda, this adaptogen was also known to foster vivid dreams and a deeper sleep. It was celebrated for its spiritual and consciousness-raising abilities.

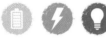

- Anxiety and depression
- Emotional/psychological stress
- Motivator

DOSAGE

Dosages differ greatly depending on usage. Consult your physician.

BENEFITS

Containing a compound known as L-dopa, the velvet bean increases dopamine in the brain, which causes an immediate mood boost. L-dopa is a precursor to dopamine, a chemical in the brain that affects movement, pleasure sensations, and emotions. This compound is also what makes it a natural aphrodisiac, increasing the sensation of pleasure. The bean is a psychoactive, just like coffee, but it's nonaddictive, unlike coffee. This adaptogen is known to increase mental clarity, reduce the feeling of emotional stress, and give an overall sense of well-being. The same compound, L-dopa, is also responsible for improving muscle growth and strength, reducing the discomfort of PMS symptoms in women and helping infertility in men.[6] In addition to its traditional use, research surrounding its benefits for those with Parkinson's disease are being studied extensively.[7]

SAFETY

This is an adaptogen that benefits from sporadic use. It is best taken one week on, one week off. When ingested, it should be taken without food. Always consult your physician before adding velvet bean to your routine.

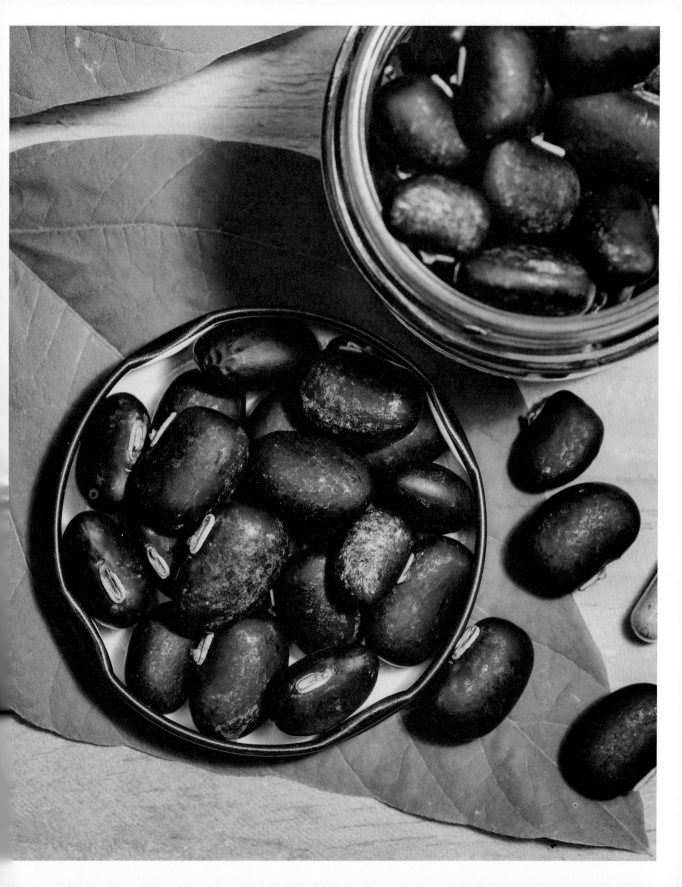

HOLY BASIL (TULSI)
OCIMUM SANCTUM

HISTORY

This superherb has been used in Ayurveda for around three thousand years. It is also considered one of India's most sacred herbs and is grown in nearly every courtyard in the country for brewing a delicious and refreshing tea. Hindus view this herb as a manifestation of Lakshmi, the goddess of wealth, love, and prosperity. They believe this plant is endowed with great spiritual powers. This herb has long been used as an expectorant for bronchitis. A natural detoxifier, it's also effective for relief of an upset stomach and as a healthy response to stress. The herb can help return our bodies to homeostasis.

- Mood enhancer
- Immune booster
- Antiviral
- Gas reliever
- Diuretic
- Expectorant
- Seasonal allergies

DOSAGE

Take 40 to 60 drops in extract form, up to three times a day, or take 1 teaspoon of the dried herb once a day.

BENEFITS

One of the main benefits of holy basil is that, unlike other adaptogens that need to build up in the body to offer benefits, this one has an immediate calming ability. This sacred herb supports the immune and digestive systems. It has been shown to lower blood pressure, help maintain ideal weight, lower cortisol levels, and treat environmental allergies and asthma with the help of its antioxidants. Holy basil is also used to restore the nervous system with mental clarity, treat minor depression, and even aid in recovering from head trauma. Spiritually, this adaptogen is used to bring the chakras back into balance.

SAFETY

Holy basil has been shown to cause infertility in men, so it's best to avoid it if you are trying to get pregnant or if you are pregnant. It is also a mild diuretic. Always consult your physician before adding it to your routine.

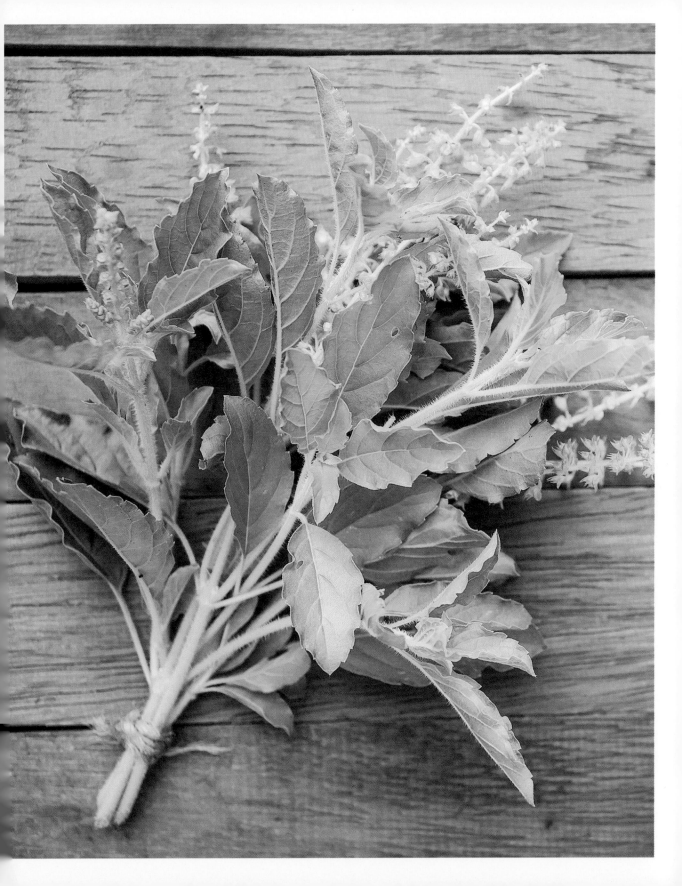

GINSENG, ASIAN
PANAX GINSENG

HISTORY

This ginseng hails from the mountainous forests of China and Korea, and, like its American counterpart, it is on the verge of extinction due to high demand. In fact, the only Asian ginseng on the market today is cultivated. This adaptogen has long been used in Traditional Chinese Medicine for longevity and stimulation.

- Immune support
- Heart health
- Levels blood sugar
- Libido enhancer for men and women
- Adrenal support

DOSAGE

Take 20 to 40 drops of extract, up to three times a day, or take 1 to 2 teaspoons of dried herb once a day.

BENEFITS

Asian ginseng is quite interesting because of its chameleon-like properties. It is one of the most stimulating ones available, but it can feel calming to those who have anxiety. Ginseng's libido-enhancing benefits for both men and women are widely known, but it has also been found to help correct memory in age-related cognitive deterioration, improve learning speed and retention, and enhance alertness.

Adrenal exhaustion is another area where Asian ginseng can work wonders. When we are run down, exhausted, and depleted, its uplifting effects can work wonders. It has been shown to help with an over- or underactive immune system and has some lovely anti-inflammatory properties.

SAFETY

Asian ginseng has been shown to cause headaches, anxiety, diarrhea, high blood pressure, and insomnia in those who are highly sensitive to it. Those on blood thinners and antidepressants should consult their physician before including it in their routine because of potential interactions. Avoid caffeine while taking Asian ginseng. Always consult your physician before adding it to your routine.

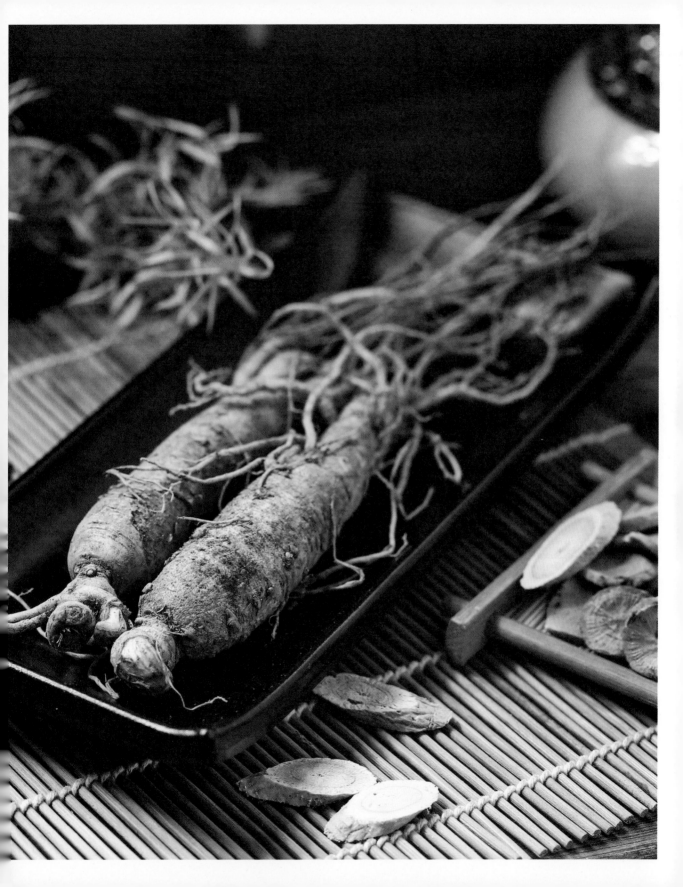

GINSENG, AMERICAN
PANAX QUINQUEFOLIUS

HISTORY

This adaptogen is probably the best known of all. It is different from its Asian namesake; in fact, they each have different medicinal properties. Although it is known for enhancing energy and the male libido, American ginseng has many other incredible benefits. This herb grows wild, mainly in North America, and is so desired that it is now on the United States endangered species list. It is most potent when mature and is often not allowed to be picked until it reaches maturity, around five to ten years old.

- Stimulates central nervous system
- Immune booster
- Stimulant
- Menopause symptoms
- Erectile dysfunction
- Athletic performance

DOSAGE

I recommend starting low and increasing dosage as you deem fit for yourself. Take 50 to 100 drops in extract form, up to three times a day, or 1 to 2 teaspoons of dried herb a day.

BENEFITS

American ginseng, although clearly a stimulant, boasts many other benefits that are often overlooked. Usages range from fighting infections, like the common cold, all the way to being included in the HIV/AIDS infection fight.[8] Some use this ginseng to aid in digestive health, loss of appetite, nausea, colitis, or gastritis. It has been shown in studies to help alleviate anemia, cancer-related fatigue, insomnia, and erectile dysfunction. Benefits enjoyed by those who take American ginseng include improved mental and athletic performance and more moderate menopausal symptoms, to name just a few.

SAFETY

American ginseng is a stimulant and may be too stimulating for some people. Headaches, diarrhea, insomnia, nervousness, rapid heart rate, high blood pressure, low blood pressure, and rash have all been reported while taking this plant. Do not take it if you are pregnant or breastfeeding. Always consult your physician before adding American ginseng to your routine.

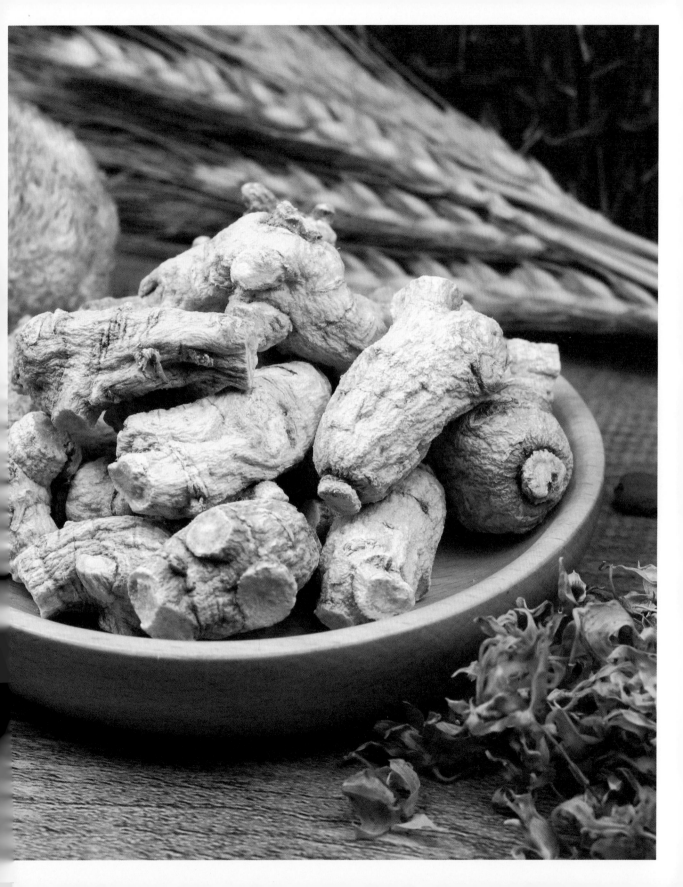

PEARL

HISTORY

This phenomenal adaptogen, literally ground-up freshwater pearls, is used in Traditional Chinese Medicine and Ayurveda practices. In TCM, the pearl was the highest-rated medicine for achieving a youthful appearance, glowing skin, and overall skin health. Pearl powder was used for outward beauty in Chinese medicine, but it was also said to alleviate stress and anxiety and create a calm disposition. Another practice, dating back millennia, found wealthy Chinese women ingesting pearl powder while pregnant to ensure that their children would have clear and glowing complexions. Most TCM practitioners state that the pearl must be combined with other medicinal ingredients and used at the proper times for these results.

In Ayurveda, this powder, known as *mukta pishti*, is used in love potions and as an aphrodisiac, as well as for anti-aging, to settle the digestion, to alleviate extra heat in the body, and to soothe inflammation.

- Hair health
- Skin health
- Nail health
- Radiance
- Strong bones

DOSAGE

Take 300 to 500 mg of powder, up to three times a day.

BENEFITS

The ancient uses for pearl powder are being proven in modern science today. The pearl contains at least 30 trace minerals. The highest doses are calcium, iron, copper, magnesium, silica, and selenium. These minerals are responsible for promoting healthy, glowing, plump, and youthful skin, as well as encouraging collagen production. They also aid in strengthening the hair, nails, and skin, and promoting healing. The calcium- and collagen-supporting benefits of this adaptogen also aid in bone, joint, to settle digestion, and recovery support. It works from the inside out to give us the universally desired glow, and it can also be applied topically to get the same benefits.

SAFETY

This powder has lots of calcium, so the dosage should not exceed what is recommended. Always consult your physician before including it in your routine. The most absorbable pearl powder is hydrolyzed and is made from pure freshwater pearls. There are many other forms of pearl powder that are of lesser quality, so be careful.

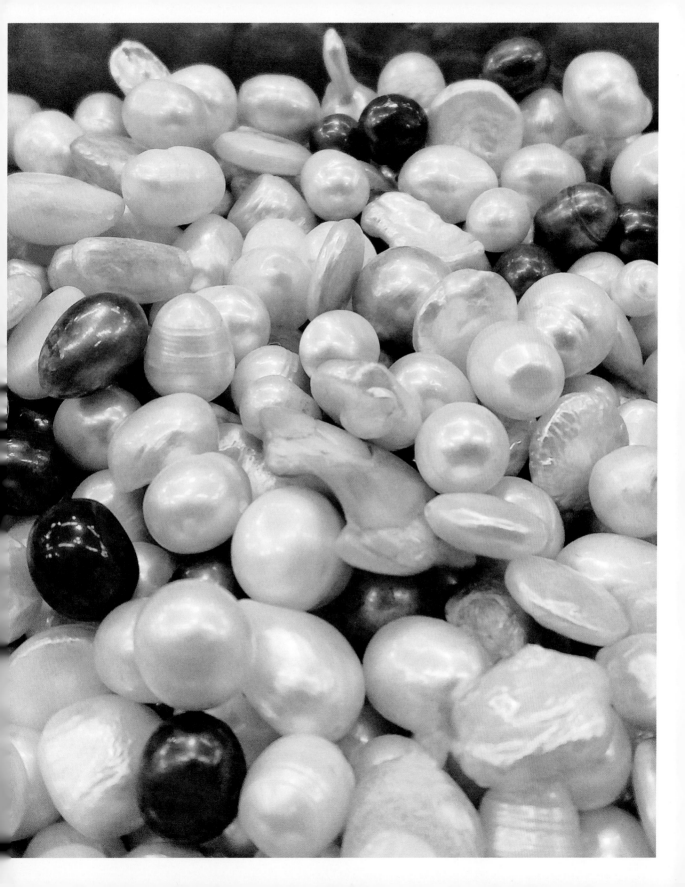

PINE POLLEN

HISTORY

Pine pollen has long been used in Traditional Chinese Medicine, with a wide variety of uses. Known to be nontoxic, this mild and sweet pollen was used to restore qi from cold and fever in the heart and abdomen. It could also help stop bleeding, aid in urination, nourish qi, give strength and energy, treat postnatal headaches, soothe an upset mood, quench thirst, create longevity, and even to make a delicious pastry!

- Aphrodisiac
- Metabolism booster
- Hormone balancing
- Immune support
- Brain boosting

DOSAGE

Pine pollen works best when absorbed through the mucous membrane in the mouth. Mix with a little water and hold it under the tongue for a few seconds before swallowing. This will ensure you receive all of its benefits. The dose of pine pollen differs greatly from extracts to pills. Review your individual goals before deciding on a dosage.

BENEFITS

Pine pollen is the only known plant source that contains the hormone DHEA, which is produced by the adrenal glands; these are the same glands that often get overworked and exhausted. As a predecessor to testosterone, estrogen, and progesterone, DHEA is responsible for increasing libido, balancing the mood, boosting immunity, and revving up our sex drive. Pine pollen is also a known antiviral and anti-inflammatory agent. It contains vitamin D3, which is hard to find in a food source. It also contains many vitamins, minerals, and amino acids. This substance is also said to help us relate back to our spiritual self and nature: as a truly wild food, it can help bring balance back to our endocrine system. Other benefits of this adaptogen include clearing acne and eczema, aiding in recovery from hangover symptoms, and lowering high cholesterol.

SAFETY

This is a pollen, so if you have allergies it might not be the right adaptogen for you. Pine pollen also contains testosterone, a hormone that needs to stay within certain levels; if these levels get too high, side-effects may occur, including blood clots in the legs, cardiovascular problems, increased risk of prostate cancer, acne, and low sperm count. Pregnant and breastfeeding women should avoid pine pollen. Always consult your physician before adding it to your routine.

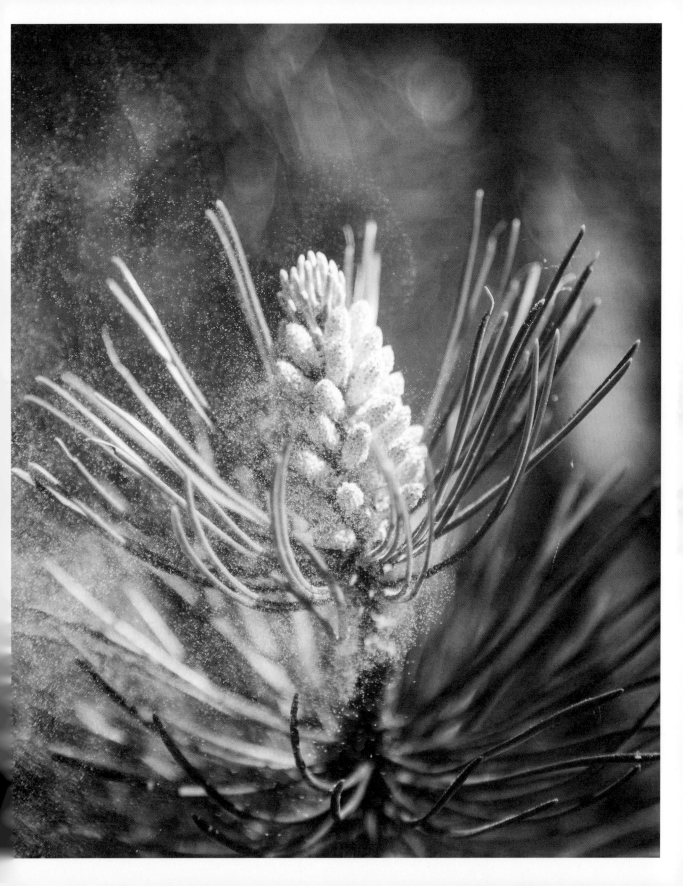

HE SHOU WU (FO-TI)
POLYGONUM MULTIFLORUM

HISTORY

The translation of this adaptogen's common name is "Black-Haired Mr. He." Mr. He was the discoverer of its properties, which included turning his grey hair back to black and helping him father a child when he believed he was sterile. Such are the bizarre folk tales surrounding this herb, and its beginning is definitely a strange one. He shou wu is also said to be a spirit tonic. Some say it brings out people's creativity and aids them in becoming more intuitive and receptive.

- Immune support
- Blood cleanser
- Laxative
- Cholesterol reducer
- Fatigue fighter
- Erectile dysfunction
- Constipation aid
- Hair health

DOSAGE

Take 30 to 40 drops of extract up to three times a day, or 1 to 2 teaspoons of dried herb, up to three times a day.

BENEFITS

He shou wu is used for many purposes today, premature graying still being one of them, though this is probably the least of its powers. This intelligent plant is also used as a longevity tonic, with its potent antioxidant capacity. It's also used to nourish the liver and kidneys, improve fatigue, ease lower back pain, aid in erectile dysfunction, help with constipation, and ease inflammation of the intestines. He shou wu has also been shown to support the immune system and calm the nervous system.

SAFETY

This herb in large doses has been known to cause diarrhea and stomach upset. He shou wu should not be combined with hepatotoxic (toxic to the liver) medications like acetaminophen, tetracycline, and statins. Always consult with your physician before adding this herb to your routine.

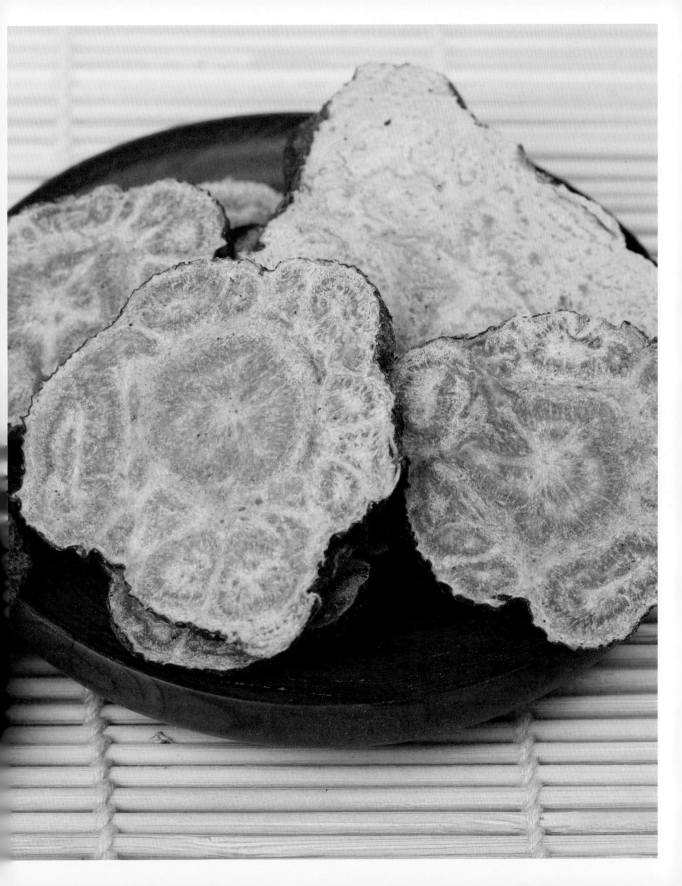

RHAPONTICUM
RHAPONTICUM CARTHAMOIDES

HISTORY

This perennial herb, also known as maral root, has been used for centuries in Siberia and eastern Europe. It was commonly combined with another adaptogen, rhodiola (see page 78). It aids in the body's healthy response to stress while also supporting sexual libido. In Traditional Chinese Medicine, this herb has been used to aid in the painful symptoms of mastitis, sores, clogged milk ducts, and swollen lymph nodes. It is known to expel heat and reduce toxic swelling.

- Stamina and endurance
- Menopause support
- Libido enhancer for men and women
- Stress reducer

DOSAGE

Dosage greatly differs depending on use, age, health, and other conditions.

BENEFITS

Today, rhaponticum is used to support mental fortitude by aiding in the stress response, promote physical stamina by delivering adequate oxygen to muscles before and during exercise, and aiding in natural resilience by supporting normal glucose levels and offering antioxidant support. This adaptogen has also been shown to support and ease women's symptoms during menopause.

SAFETY

Rhaponticum is not to be used while pregnant. Only use during breastfeeding when working with a licensed herbalist. Always consult with your physician before including it in your routine.

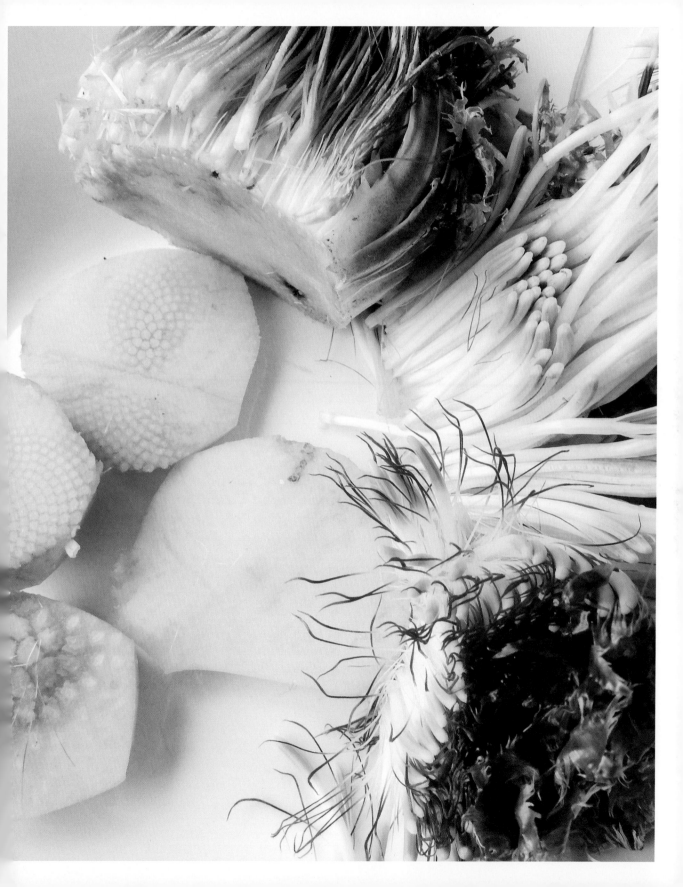

RHODIOLA
RHODIOLA ROSEA

HISTORY

This succulent, also known as the "golden root," is one that grows in the most frigid conditions, making it a hearty, resilient, and thriving plant. Originally found in northern Asia, Canada, Russia, and the Scandinavian countries, this intelligent plant was first used to increase mental and physical stamina and endurance. When consumed regularly, it was used to help prevent illness in the coldest, darkest months. In fact, emperors in China sent their constituents on expeditions to Siberia in search of rhodiola, from which they created a tonic to treat colds and flu. In Siberia, this herb was brewed into a tea and given to newlyweds to boost their fertility and increase their chances of having a healthy baby.

- Endurance and stamina
- Memory enhancer
- Clarity
- Anxiety and depression
- Fatigue fighter

DOSAGE

Take 40 to 60 drops of extract up to three times a day, or dried herb, 1 to 2 teaspoons, up to three times a day.

BENEFITS

This plant is known as an athlete's best friend. During hard training, our immune systems take a beating: this herb has been shown to support the immune system, strengthen physical performance, and shorten recovery time. The perfect example of a chameleon, rhodiola has a balancing effect: when the body needs emotional calm, it aids in lowering cortisol levels; when it needs cerebral stimulation, rhodiola helps increase mental clarity and memory function. This plant has been shown to normalize blood sugar, decrease exhaustion symptoms, and offer both aphrodisiac and antidepressant effects. It also has an amazing ability to increase serotonin to help regulate sleep, mood, and appetite.

SAFETY

It's best to take rhodiola early in the day; when taken too late, it can cause insomnia. Some studies have shown that this adaptogen does not function properly if you have mental health issues.[9] Always consult with your physician before adding it to your routine.

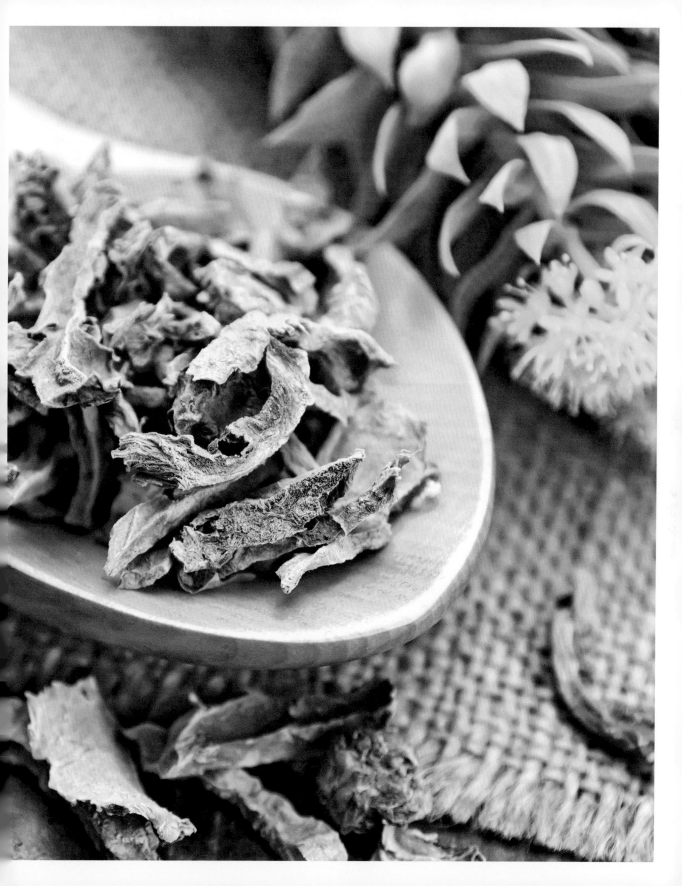

ELDERBERRY
SAMBUCUS NIGRA

HISTORY

The elderberry and elderflower have a longstanding relationship in both fiction and nonfiction. In certain myths, the elder tree was used to ward off witches, while others claim that witches chose elder woods for their meetings. Vampires can be fended off when elder wood is made into a stake, according to legend. In the British Isles, bathing your eyes in elder juice could allow you to see fairies. It's even used in the Harry Potter novels as the best wood for making a wand. In reality, the elderberry has a long history in Traditional Chinese Medicine. A medicinal wine made from the berries can be used to treat rheumatism as well as the pain from traumatic injuries.

- Cold and flu buster
- Immune support
- Blood pressure
- Skin health

DOSAGE

Because there are so many forms of elderberry on the market, each has a different dosage. Lozenges, syrups, and teas are common forms of this adaptogen. Look for one without added sweeteners or sugars.

BENEFITS

Along with other berries, the elderberry is rich in antioxidants, vitamin C, vitamin A, vitamin B6, iron, potassium, and fiber. Before you pick some elderberries, you should know that they're poisonous if eaten raw, so only ingest cooked products of these berries.

In syrup form, they are used to treat everything from the common cold to the flu. In some studies, elderberry has been shown to support overall immune health, and it can also level out your blood pressure. On the outside, this berry has also been shown to improve skin health. With its rich source of antioxidants, it can support collagen, prevent wrinkles, fight inflammation, and even overall tone and softness—all reasons to include it in your routine.

SAFETY

Again, raw elderberries are not to be consumed because of their toxic levels of cyanide-releasing compounds. If pregnant or breastfeeding, it's a good idea to stay away from elderberry. It is also possible that those with autoimmune diseases should not include this berry in their diets, as the elderberry might cause an overstimulation of the immune system. Always consult your physician before adding it to your routine.

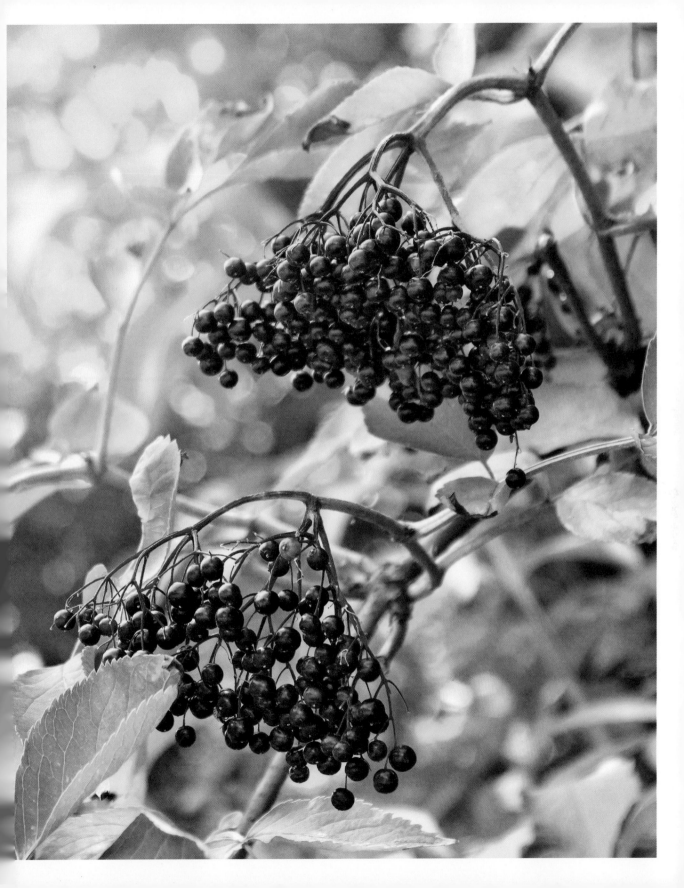

SCHISANDRA BERRY
SCHISANDRA CHINENSIS

HISTORY

This plant's berries are the medicinal part of the vine. In Chinese, the name is translated as "fruit of the five flavors:" when you hold the berry in your mouth for a few minutes and chew, it reveals its many layers. The peel is sweet, sour, and a little salty, then, upon further tasting, the seeds become bitter in flavor. In Traditional Chinese Medicine, this berry was used to balance the yin and yang. In Russia, a tea tonic was made to fight fatigue. Additionally, this adaptogen has been used to dry excessive fluids. It is beneficial in the treatment of diarrhea, wet coughs, frequent urination, and reproductive problems such as premature ejaculation and excessive vaginal discharge.

- Skin health
- Immunity
- Endurance and strength
- Anxiety

DOSAGE

Take 40 to 80 drops in extract, up to four times a day, or 1 to 2 teaspoons of dried herb up to three times a day.

BENEFITS

The schisandra berry is a great source of vitamin C, as well as providing an overall balancing effect for the endocrine system. That is why taking it at times of high stress can be incredibly beneficial, because it supports the immune system and backs it up with antioxidants. This intelligent plant knows if you need help in raising your blood pressure or lowering it, and it acts accordingly, stabilizing and nourishing the blood and its pressure. It can also help enhance reflexes and concentration while helping relieve anxiety.

SAFETY

This adaptogen is not suitable during pregnancy or while breastfeeding. Some studies have found that the schisandra berry increases stomach acid, so it should be avoided if you have ulcers or gastritis. It is also not suitable during acute illnesses. Always consult your physician before adding it to your routine.

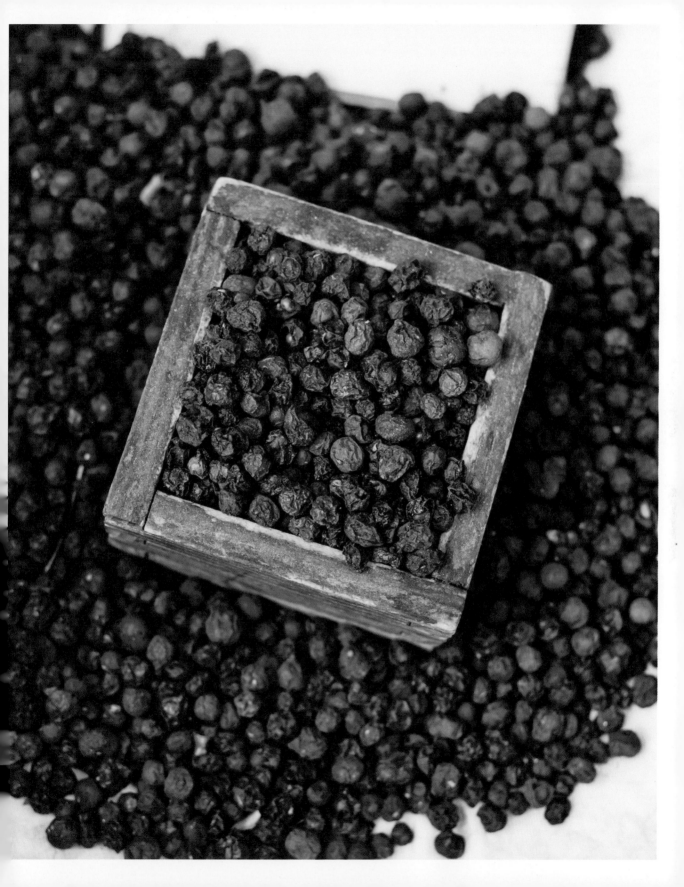

SHILAJIT

HISTORY

Shilajit, also known as mineral pitch, is the result of a long process of breaking down plant matter and minerals. The result is a sticky, black, tarlike substance derived from rocks in high mountain ranges. This compound has been used in Ayurvedic medicine for centuries as a rejuvenating tonic and an aphrodisiac.

- Overall health and well-being
- Cognitive improvement
- Male hormone health
- Fatigue fighter
- Anti-aging
- Fertility

DOSAGE

Take 300 to 500 mg of extract, one to three times a day, or 1 to 2 teaspoons of dried tar one to three times a day.

BENEFITS

There is quite a roster of benefits associated with shilajit. The first, also the most studied, is its effect on Alzheimer's disease: the molecular composition of shilajit is believed to slow or even possibly prevent the progression of this form of dementia. The antioxidant in the substance, known as fulvic acid, is a great contributor to cognitive health. Tau proteins are an important part of our nervous system, but they can prompt brain cell damage when they build up. Shilajit helps prevent the accumulation of tau protein. Shilajit can also increase testosterone levels in men. Low testosterone is a common male ailment and contributes to a low sex drive, hair loss, loss of muscle mass, fatigue, and increased body fat. Other benefits of shilajit include combating chronic fatigue syndrome, and it's a versatile anti-inflammatory, aiding in slowing the premature aging process, helping with iron-deficiency, reversing male infertility, and improving heart health.

SAFETY

Make sure you are buying shilajit from a reputable manufacturer. The product should be processed prior to being consumed: raw, unprocessed shilajit may contain contaminants that could make you sick. It is also important to avoid this adaptogen if you have sickle-cell anemia or too much iron in your blood. Always consult with your physician before adding it to your routine.

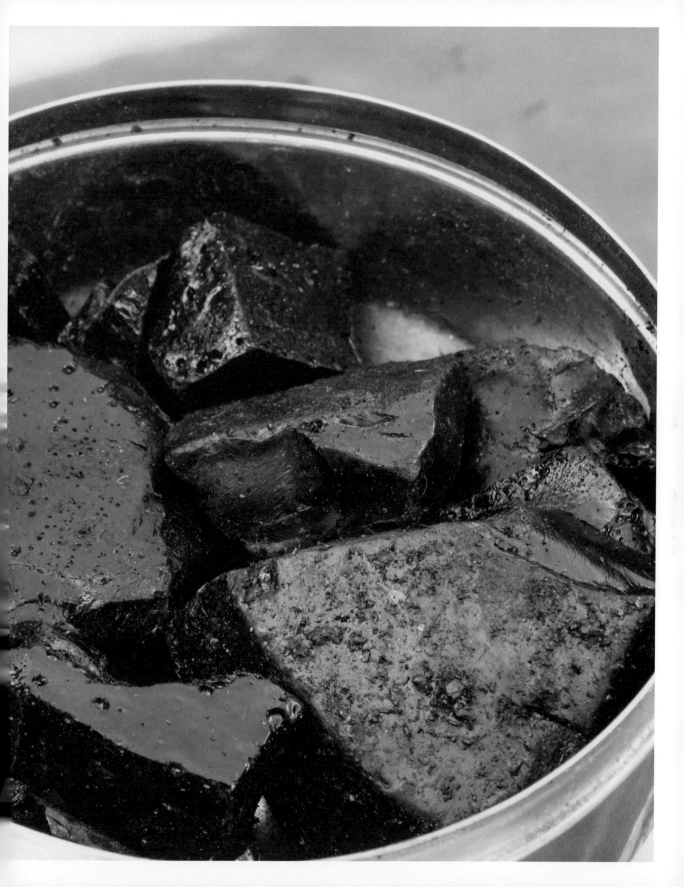

GUDUCHI
TINOSPORA CORDIFOLIA

HISTORY

This plant is highly regarded in Ayurvedic medicine. It is known as the "heavenly elixir," "nectar of life," and "one that protects the body." Guduchi is traditionally used as an internal and external toxin remover to promote longevity, increase strength and appetite, and ease skin issues, as well as for its aphrodisiac, blood purification, and digestive aid properties.

- Toxin remover
- Longevity
- Aphrodisiac
- Immune booster
- Allergy sufferers

DOSAGE

Take 3 to 6 g of the dried herb up to two times a day.

BENEFITS

Guduchi has beneficial immune-boosting qualities. When this adaptogen is added into one's daily routine, studies have found that the body's immune system is able to rid itself of harmful microbes, bacteria, and other harmful substances. This herb is also beneficial for liver health. Some studies have shown that this herb has the ability to reverse damage done to the liver from alcoholism by improving functions and regulating antioxidant enzymes, cholesterol activity, and liver enzyme activity. Guduchi is also particularly effective in aiding allergy symptoms. Stuffy nose, sneezing, and itching are significantly decreased with this herb's addition to your routine. Other benefits include detoxification, due to its potent antioxidant content. It has a proven ability to lower blood sugar, treat rheumatic disorders, and offer general rejuvenation.

SAFETY

Guduchi has been shown to cause stomach upset when taken in large quantities over long periods of time. This herb is not safe to take while pregnant or breastfeeding. Always consult with your physician before adding it to your routine.

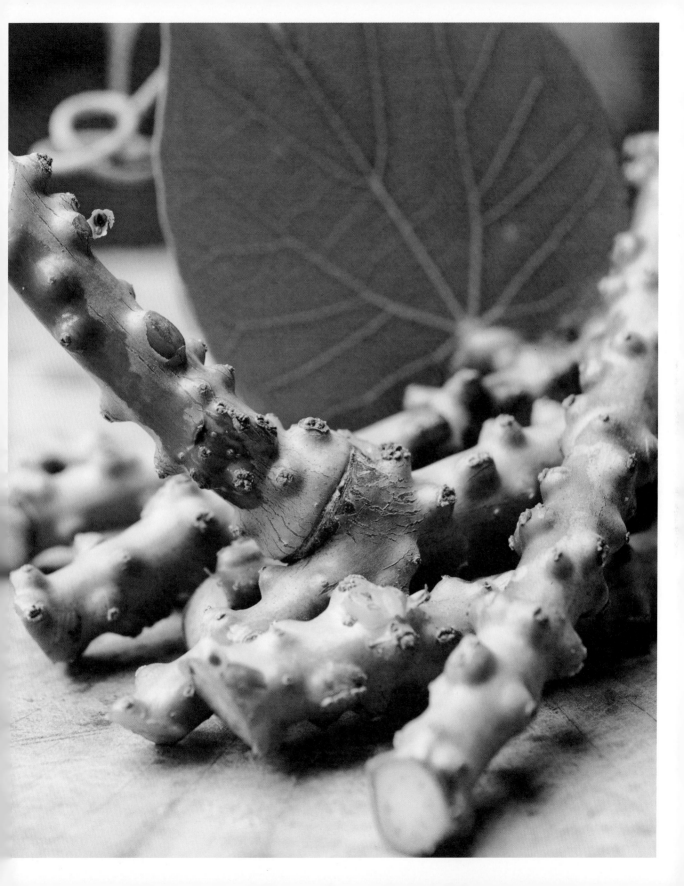

TURKEY TAIL
TRAMETES VERSICOLOR

HISTORY

This mushroom, found throughout Traditional Chinese Medicine as well as in Japanese medicine, was often called the "cloud mushroom." Traditionally, the turkey tail mushroom was used as a tea tonic, offering beneficial properties for the spirit, qi, or vital energy, while also strengthening the bones and tendons. In the 1960s, both China and Japan began using the extract of this mushroom to treat various cancers. Since then, this mushroom has become one of the most extensively researched mushrooms to date.

- Flu fighter
- Disease fighter
- Prebiotic for gut health

DOSAGE

Dosages differ greatly depending on usage. Consult your physician.

BENEFITS

Turkey tail has wide-reaching immune support capabilities. It has long been used as a way to enhance the body's resilience to infection and illnesses. This mushroom has shown great aid in those undergoing chemotherapy, offering beneficial compounds that, when used in tandem with certain treatments, may enhance their efficacy. Turkey tail is also a prebiotic, offering dietary fiber that feeds the beneficial bacteria of the gut, creating healthy digestion and decreasing bloat. As an animal lover, I must mention one last incredible benefit of this mushroom: turkey tail is also being used in dogs to help support their immune systems and balance their gut health.

SAFETY

This mushroom is not suitable for those who are pregnant or breastfeeding. It is best to buy this adaptogen from a reputable source. Do not gather it yourself. Always consult your physician before adding this adaptogen to your routine.

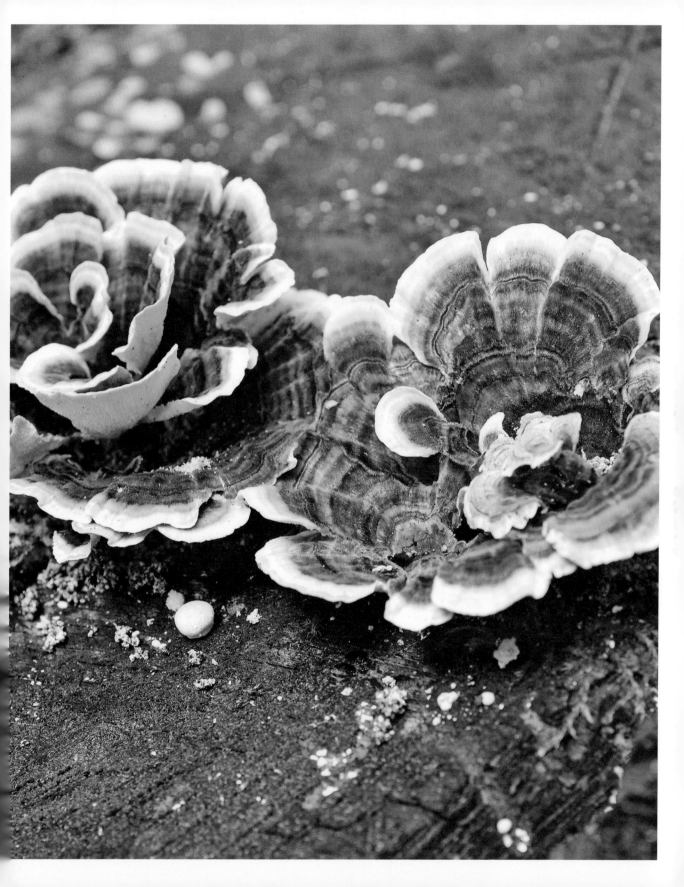

NETTLE
URTICA DIOICA

HISTORY

The stinging nettle has a long history in folk medicine. It is a flowering plant native to northern Africa, North America, Asia, and Europe. It is well named, as most hikers and gardeners can attest: skin or mucosal contact with this plant often causes a stinging sensation.

The nettle seeds have long been used in Traditional Chinese Medicine to encourage prostate and kidney health. The nutritious leaves are known to support lung, kidney, and immune health.

- Kidney health
- Adrenal health
- Immune support
- Nutrition powerhouse
- Allergy support
- Expectorant
- Circulation
- PMS

DOSAGE

The entirety of this plant can be used. For the seeds, 1 to 2 tablespoons can be added to soups and stews; eat such a dish only once a day.

Take an extract (1 to 5 drops) up to three times a day.

Fresh leaves may be used without an upper limit each day.

BENEFITS

Nettle is high in iron and protein, rich in chlorophyll, and contain a great deal of vitamins A, B1, B2, C, and K, as well as copper, calcium, and magnesium. The leaves are known for astringent, diuretic, antiallergenic, stimulating, and decongestant properties. The leaves can aid in lowering blood pressure and are used for their expectorant and antispasmodic effects. The high iron content alleviates menstrual cramps and heavy bleeding. It has long been used to dissolve of kidney stones, aids in blood clotting, and stimulate blood circulation. As a tonic it restores homeostasis to the liver, kidneys, immune system, and detoxifies the body and blood.

Nettle leaves, although packing a "sting," are also packed with nutrition. The sting is a combination of acetylcholine and formic acid, and these two reduce inflammation; improve circulation, cellular responses, and capillary stimulation and lymph flow; and even aiding in the alleviation of arthritis pain.

SAFETY

This adaptogen will cause skin irritation if touched when fresh. The application of the leaves is said to alleviate the pain. Some note stomach irritation and sweating when taking it for long periods. Do not use during pregnancy or while breastfeeding. It has been shown to decrease blood sugar levels, so use caution if you are diabetic. The nettle has also been shown to lower blood pressure, so use caution if you are prone to low blood pressure. If you have kidney problems, avoid the above-ground portions of this plant, as they are said to increase urine flow. Always consult your physician before adding nettle to your routine.

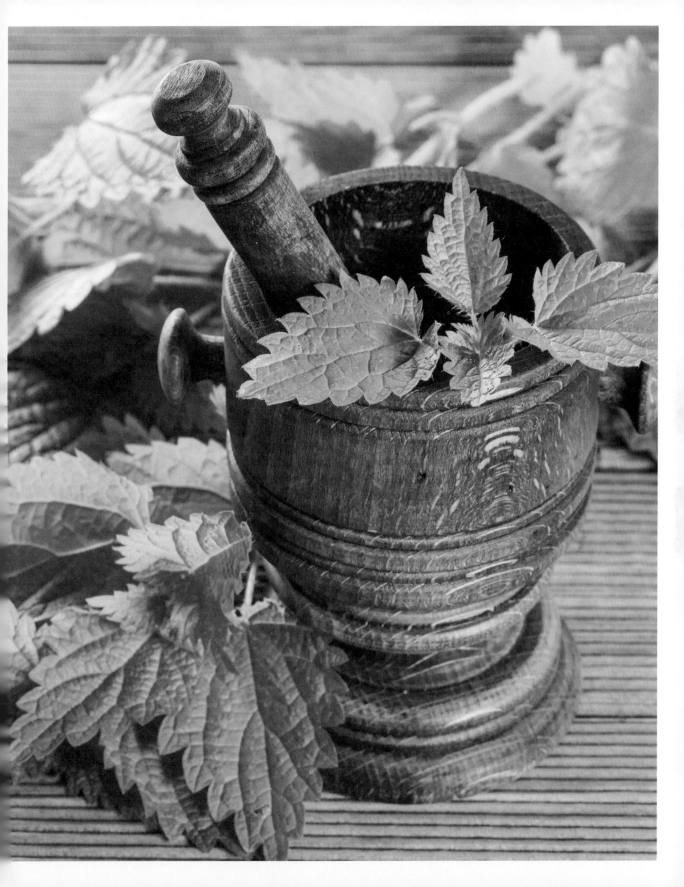

BILBERRY
(EUROPEAN BLUEBERRIES)
VACCINIUM MYRTILLUS

HISTORY

The bilberry is native to northern Europe and is often called the European blueberry because of its comparable likeness to the North American blueberry. From typhoid fever to kidney stones, this little berry has been used in many different forms. It is even said that, during World War II, the berry was made into a jam and British pilots ate it prior to flying; they claimed that it improved their night vision significantly.

- Circulation
- Antidiarrheal
- Eye health
- Allergies

DOSAGE

Differs between extracts, teas, and berries, though most range from 160 to 200 mg taken up to two times daily.

BENEFITS

This powerful antioxidant berry has been shown to strengthen blood vessels and capillary walls, improve red blood cells, and increase retinal pigments that allow the eyes to tolerate light, improving overall eyesight.[10] Just like the British pilots, adding this adaptogen to your routine can improve your night vision, while also helping slow macular degeneration, prevent cataracts, and aid in recovery from diabetic retinopathy. It has been shown to be an antifungal, antibacterial, anti-inflammatory, and antihistamine. It can kill or inhibit the growth of fungi, yeasts, and bacteria and help with atherosclerosis, bruising, poor circulation, diabetes, diarrhea, and varicose veins.

SAFETY

It is not safe to take bilberries while pregnant or breastfeeding. The leaf also has the tendency to lower blood sugar, so if you have low blood sugar or are on medications that lower your blood sugar, monitor closely. Always consult your physician before adding it to your routine.

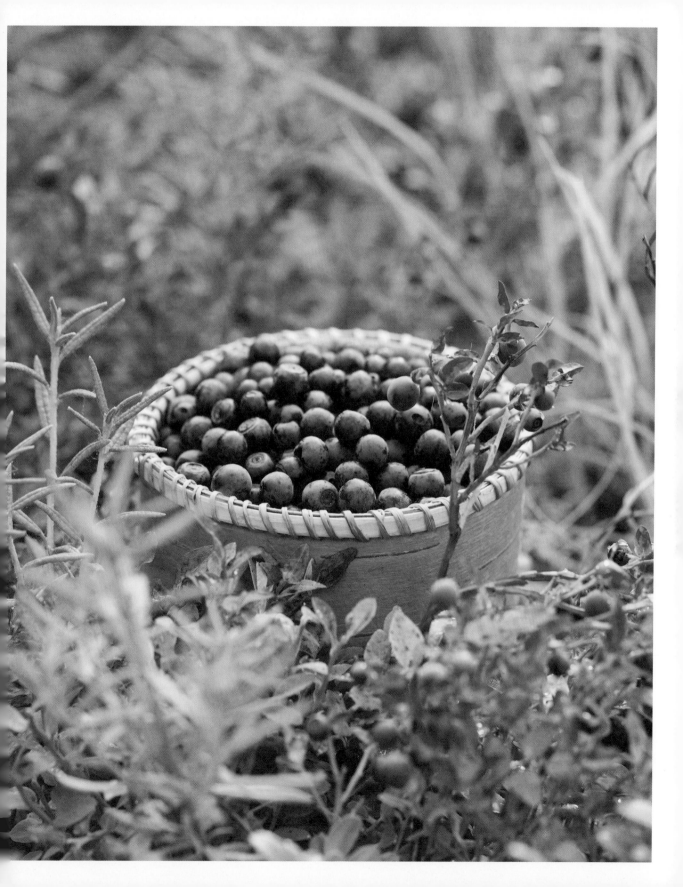

ASHWAGANDHA
WITHANIA SOMNIFERA

HISTORY

This adaptogen has been around for thousands of years in Ayurveda. It is a go-to medicine to support the immune system, used for its revitalizing properties. Ashwagandha is truly well rounded: it's great to overcome modern-day stressors and to help improve sexual health and encourage restful sleep.

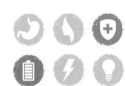

- New mom support
- Sleep problems
- Calming agent
- Immunity booster
- Fertility tonic

DOSAGE

Take 30 to 40 drops of extract, up to three times a day, or ½ teaspoon in 8 ounces of water up to three times a day.

BENEFITS

When ashwagandha is taken regularly, it has been shown to increase energy, vitality, and fortitude. This intelligent plant can stabilize our hormonal system or endocrine system by regulating the stress hormone cortisol. It is actually the only adaptogen that is known to have an invigorating effect on the thyroid gland.

In fact, ashwagandha is known for new mom support. It can help reduce the effect of stress on the body. If you're feeling tired, overwhelmed, or run down, it has an uncanny ability to support normal energy levels and regulate sleep patterns. It has also long been used in Ayurveda for lactation support and to benefit that combination known as "mom brain," which causes that unfocused, forgetful feeling.

Studies have also found that ashwagandha has the capacity to strengthen the immune system. In today's world of deadlines and constant work stressors, high blood pressure, insomnia, or chronic fatigue syndrome, everyone could benefit from taking a daily dose of ashwagandha. This adaptogen with its high dose of iron is great for those with anemia. It is also a nice source of antioxidants to help protect our bodies from oxidative stress.

SAFETY

A few groups of people should avoid ashwagandha: those who are pregnant, those who are allergic to the nightshade family, those who are on immunosuppressive therapy, those taking sedatives, and those with ulcers. In Africa, ashwagandha has traditionally been used to cause miscarriages. Since there's not enough information on its effects during pregnancy, it is best avoided by pregnant women. As a member of the nightshade family, this herb should not be taken if you have a sensitivity to this group of plants. Always consult your physician before adding it to your routine.

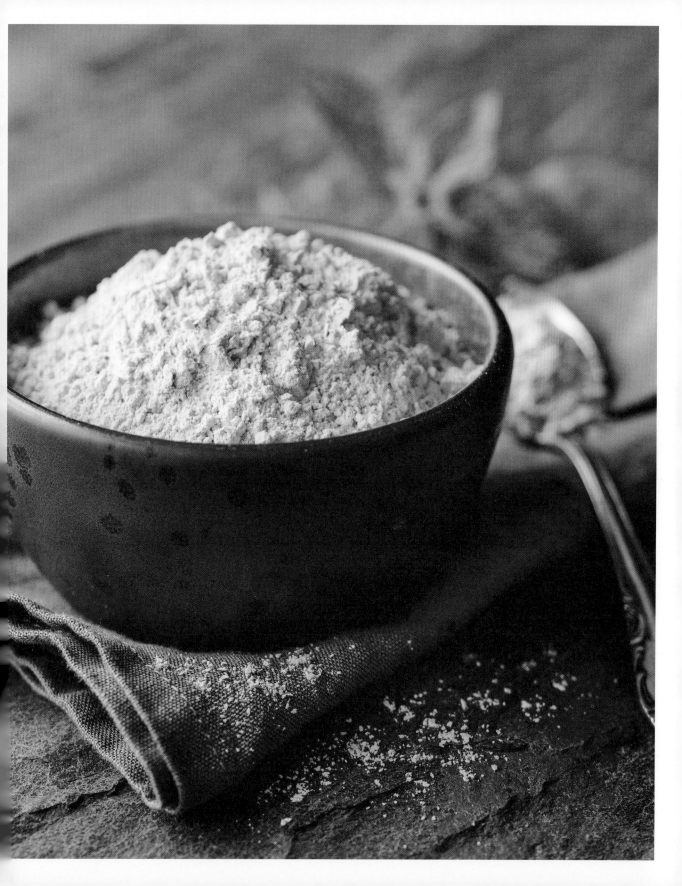

OTHER SUPERPOWDERS

The foods listed below aren't considered adaptogens in the strict sense, but I believe they are extremely special and worth mentioning. Each one is chock-full of vitamins, nutrients, antioxidants—and even superpowers. I love taking them along with adaptogens for a boost of holistic wellness. They are easy to find online or in your local health food store and are really easy to add to smoothies, teas, tonics, lattes, cookies, or other treats.

BEET

This simple-yet-super root vegetable is a powerhouse of vitamins and minerals. This root contains protein, fiber, vitamin C, vitamin B6, folate, magnesium, potassium, manganese, and iron. The rich color of beets is a great source of healthy nitrates—the bad ones are found in heavily processed meats, while the good ones are from plant sources and can help protect your heart—and antioxidants. Eating a beet is great for you, but when you add beetroot powder to your routine, the concentration of all those incredible vitamins, minerals, antioxidants, and nitrates is much higher. For instance, one teaspoon of beetroot powder is equivalent to one whole beet. Beetroot powder benefits include lowering your blood pressure, boosting brain power, fighting inflammation, stimulating healthy blood flow, supporting liver health, removing toxins from the body, improving athletic performance, and speeding up muscle recovery—just to name a few.

BUTTERFLY PEA FLOWER POWDER

This plant is discussed in Traditional Chinese Medicine and Ayurveda. It's been consumed for centuries and used to enhance memory and brain power, reduce anxiety, and as a calming agent. Butterfly pea flower powder is also used to help with premature hair loss, poor eyesight, constipation, fertility issues, and insomnia, and can be used to produce collagen. This beautiful indigo powder is rich in antioxidants, flavonoids, and peptides. Its color can also be used as a natural dye.

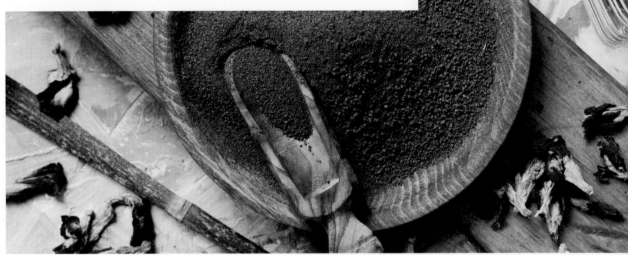

BLUE SPIRULINA

This brilliantly blue extract comes from spirulina, a freshwater algae. It is a powerful antioxidant that serves as a great source of iron, magnesium, potassium, B vitamins, and immune-boosting chlorophyll. The algae is also an anti-inflammatory and has been shown to prevent the release of histamines, which is awesome for allergy sufferers. Spirulina is a superfood that helps increase energy, strength, and endurance.

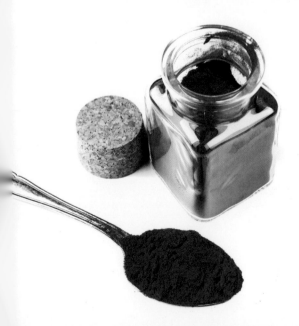

CANNABIDIOL (CBD)

I can't do this section without mentioning one of my favorite additions to anyone's daily routine. CBD is one of many cannabinoids found in the cannabis plant. Unlike THC, CBD is not a psychoactive, which means that it will not alter your perceptions when taken. This chameleon-like substance is miraculous, in that it does for the body exactly what the body needs, whether that be a natural pain reliever, an anti-inflammatory agent, an aid to help with drug withdrawal symptoms, a treatment for epilepsy or cancer, a support for anxiety disorders, a treatment for acne, or a treatment for Alzheimer's disease. Do you see how great and varied this little plant is? I am always amazed by its ability to treat such a wide variety of ailments.

CACAO POWDER

This raw, unprocessed product is what you get before processing the seed-pods of the cacao (sometimes called cocoa) tree. This antioxidant-rich powder can improve your memory, boost your mood, protect your heart, and prevent cardiovascular disease. It can be used to improve blood circulation, prevent premature aging, increase energy, lower the feeling of fatigue, create stronger hair, skin, and nails, and help lower blood pressure.

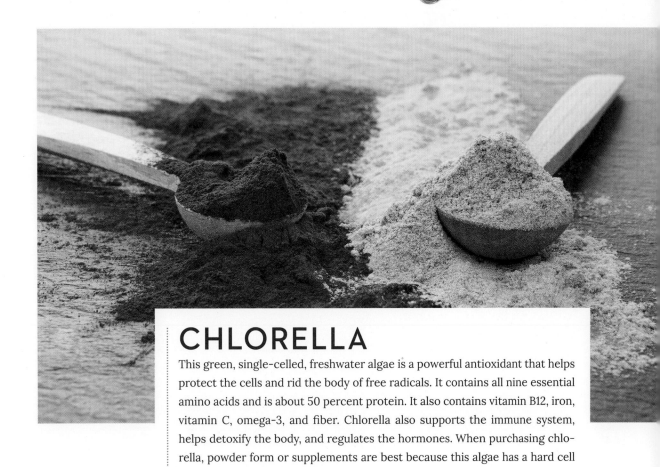

CHLORELLA

This green, single-celled, freshwater algae is a powerful antioxidant that helps protect the cells and rid the body of free radicals. It contains all nine essential amino acids and is about 50 percent protein. It also contains vitamin B12, iron, vitamin C, omega-3, and fiber. Chlorella also supports the immune system, helps detoxify the body, and regulates the hormones. When purchasing chlorella, powder form or supplements are best because this algae has a hard cell wall that is indigestible to humans.

MATCHA

This increasingly popular tea is a powerhouse of antioxidants, phytonutrients, vitamin C, vitamin E, selenium, chromium, zinc, and magnesium. Its traditional use is based on the Japanese tea ceremony, which centers on the preparation, serving, and drinking of the hot tea, encompassing a meditative spiritual style. Matcha boosts metabolism and burns calories, naturally detoxifies the body, and eases the mind and body. It contains fiber and chlorophyll, and is known to enhance concentration, lower cholesterol and blood sugar. That's quite a tea!

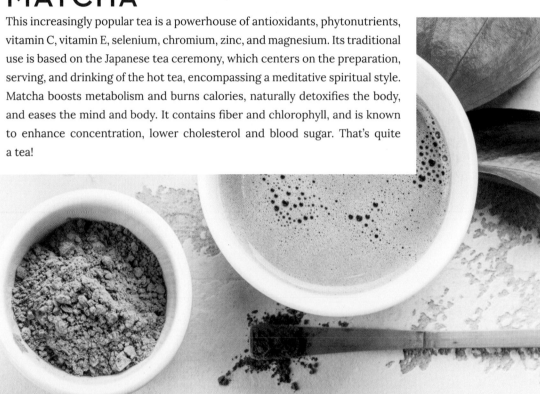

CINNAMON

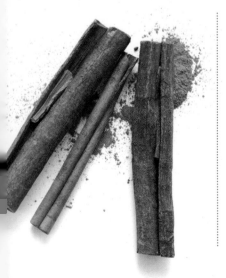

Cinnamon has been used as a spice and medicine for thousands of years. Although it started as a rare and valuable spice available only to kings, it is now widely available and inexpensive. Cinnamon contains a compound known as cinnamaldehyde, a compound useful for its health benefits. As an antioxidant powerhouse, it contains more polyphenols than garlic and oregano. It's also a great anti-inflammatory agent, with the potential to reduce the risk of heart disease by lowering total levels of cholesterol, increase sensitivity to the hormone insulin, lower blood sugar levels, function as a natural antibacterial and antifungal, and provide natural immune-boosting properties.

NOTE: Cinnamon may interfere with blood-thinning medications. Always consult your doctor before adding this to your routine.

OREGANO

This fragrant herb is often used in cooking, but it is also an effective medicine. The oil can be consumed or applied to the skin, and it is a natural antibiotic and antifungal. Oregano can help lower cholesterol levels and aids in weight loss. This powerful antioxidant helps to protect the body from damage caused by free radicals. As an oil, it has also been proven to treat one of the most common yeast infections that occurs today, candida, a yeast associated with some gut illnesses such as Crohn's disease and ulcerative colitis. Oregano oil has been shown to improve gut health by killing parasites and bad bacteria; it's also an anti-inflammatory agent.

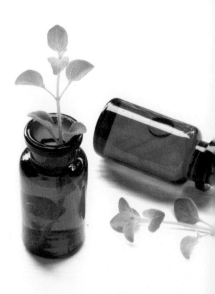

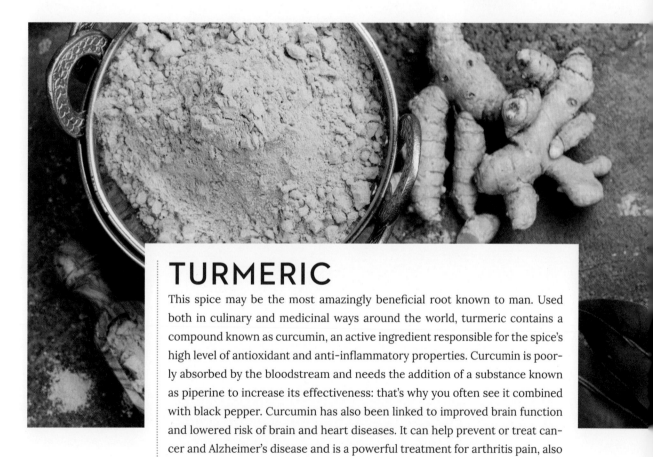

TURMERIC

This spice may be the most amazingly beneficial root known to man. Used both in culinary and medicinal ways around the world, turmeric contains a compound known as curcumin, an active ingredient responsible for the spice's high level of antioxidant and anti-inflammatory properties. Curcumin is poorly absorbed by the bloodstream and needs the addition of a substance known as piperine to increase its effectiveness: that's why you often see it combined with black pepper. Curcumin has also been linked to improved brain function and lowered risk of brain and heart diseases. It can help prevent or treat cancer and Alzheimer's disease and is a powerful treatment for arthritis pain, also serving to treat depression and aid in all-round longevity.

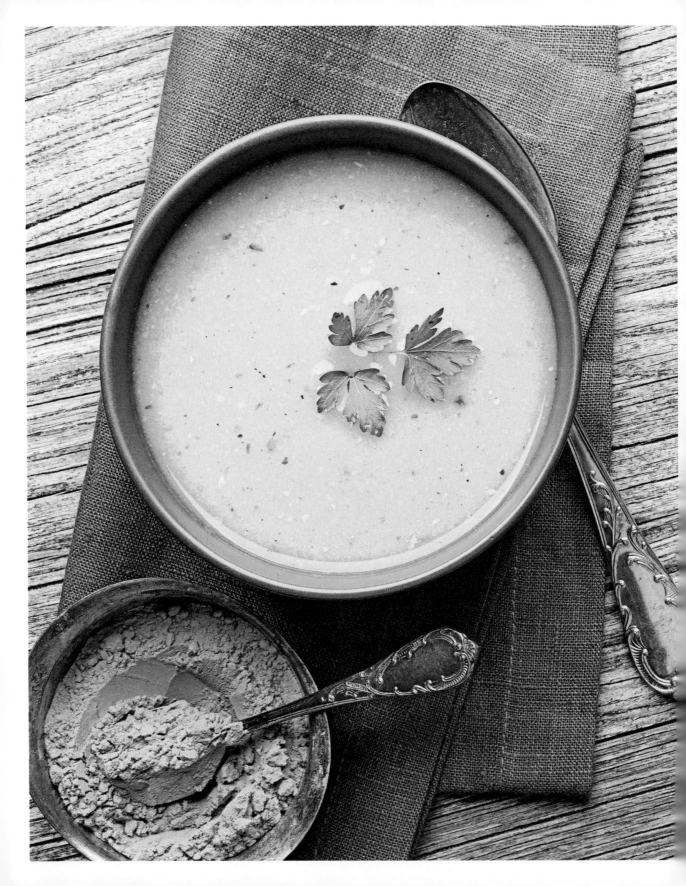

RECIPES

The following recipes are ways to incorporate adaptogens into your daily routine through mindful eating and drinking. All the plants in this book are meant to be consumed with intention, using your five senses to fully allow them to nourish your mind, body, and soul. Sometimes taking them in pill form is easiest, but when you consume them through a latte, a soup, a pudding, or a truffle, you get to fully be present and savor them in that moment. Each recipe is also linked back to our wellness icons (see page 19), making them easy to pick and choose for what you are looking for: stress reduction, skin health, digestion, mental clarity, immunity boosts, and/or energy levels. Enjoy and savor!

GLOW CHAI

 Healing, Resilience, Glow-from-Within, Hormone Balance

Traditional chai is warming, comforting, and invigorating, all in one beautiful teacup. This chai can help enhance your skin, with chaga mushrooms creating the base for resilience and healing, pearl for that glow-from-within power, maca for hormone balance, and rhodiola for clarity and strength.

INGREDIENTS

1 cup (2.4 dl) filtered water

3 grams chaga mushroom powder

1-inch (2.5 cm) fresh piece of ginger root, peeled sliced

4 cardamom pods, smashed

5 whole cloves

1 cinnamon stick

1 pod star anise

¼ tspn pearl powder

½ tbsp black peppercorns

1 cup (2.4 dl) coconut milk

¼ tspn maca

¼ tspn rhodiola

1 tspn coconut nectar

DIRECTIONS

1. Place the water, chaga powder, fresh ginger and all the spices up to the black peppercorns in a small saucepan. Warm over low heat, making sure never to let the mixture boil. Simmer for 30 minutes.

2. Add the coconut milk, maca, rhodiola, and coconut nectar to the mixture and stir to incorporate.

3. Strain into a mug and sip to enjoy!

MAKES ONE SERVING

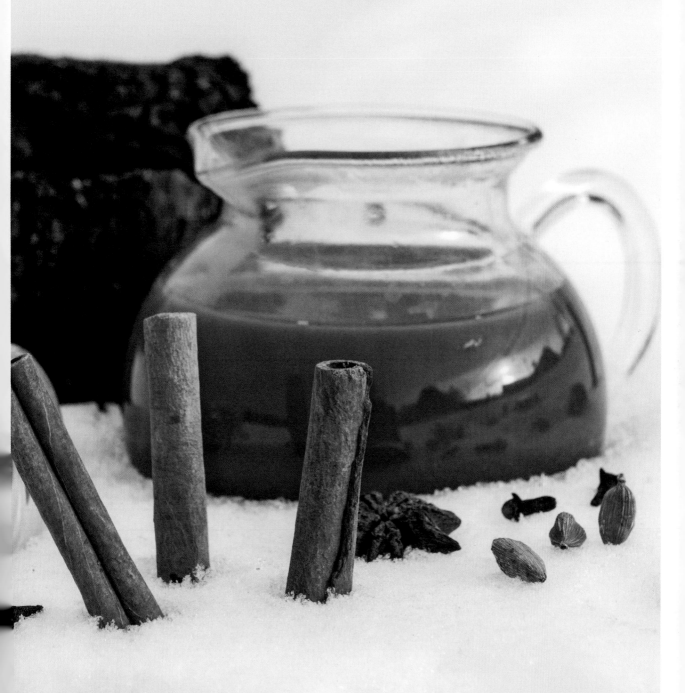

MATCHA FOCUS LATTE

 Focus, Stamina, Energizer, Immune Booster

Matcha is a great alternative to coffee. I love this one hot, but it can also be made with cold milk in an iced version. The combination of matcha and moringa makes it a beverage full of antioxidants, vitamins, minerals, and chlorophyll. The addition of CBD makes it a perfect, anxiety-free start to your day!

INGREDIENTS

2 tspn matcha powder

1 tspn moringa leaf powder

1 tspn cordyceps

¼ tspn velvet bean

¼ cup (0.6 dl) warm water

1 cup (2.4 dl) hemp
or coconut milk, warmed

1 tspn coconut nectar
or maple syrup

1 to 2 drops full-spectrum
CBD oil

DIRECTIONS

1. In a mug, whisk together the matcha, moringa, cordyceps, and velvet bean with the warm water. Whisk well until there are no lumps.

2. Whisk in the warm milk of your choice, coconut nectar, or maple syrup and CBD oil. Enjoy!

MAKES ONE SERVING

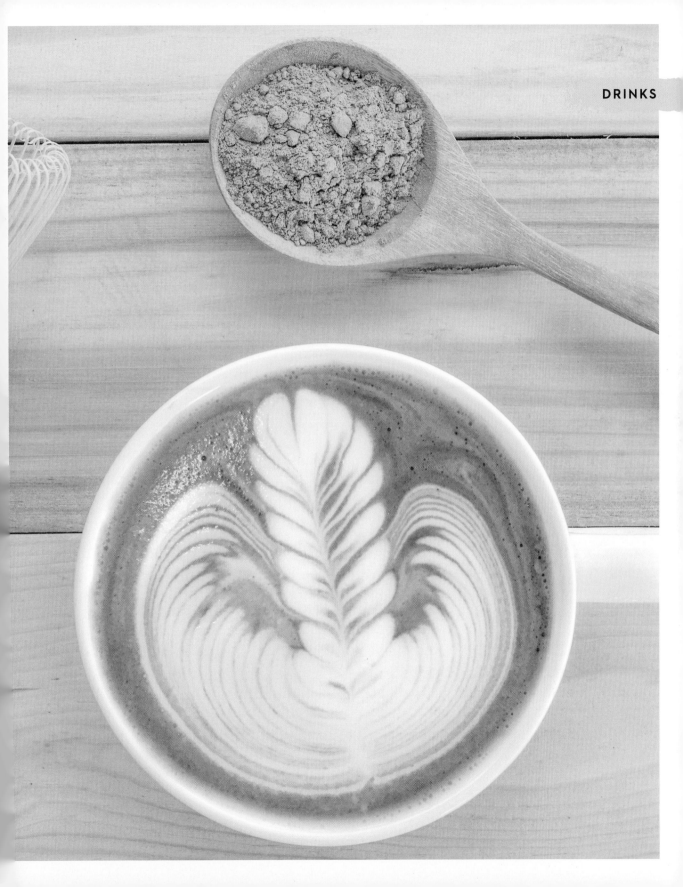

COAT-MY-THROAT LICORICE LATTE

 Respiratory Nourishment, Cooling, Digestion

This licorice, rosehip latte is a great one if you're running hot and need
to cool down, if you have excessive mucus, or if you have dry skin.
The combination of licorice and rosehip is lightly hypnotic and calming.

INGREDIENTS

1 cup (2.4 dl) water

½ tspn rosehips

¼ tspn licorice root powder

1 tspn maple syrup

¼ cup (0.6 dl) unsweetened
cashew milk

DIRECTIONS

1. Over high heat, bring the water to a boil in a small saucepan. Add
in the rosehips and licorice root powder, turn off the heat, cover,
and steep for 10 minutes.

2. Strain the liquid into your favorite mug, stir in the maple syrup.

3. Add in the cashew milk and froth with a frother for 1 minute.
Enjoy!

MAKES ONE SERVING

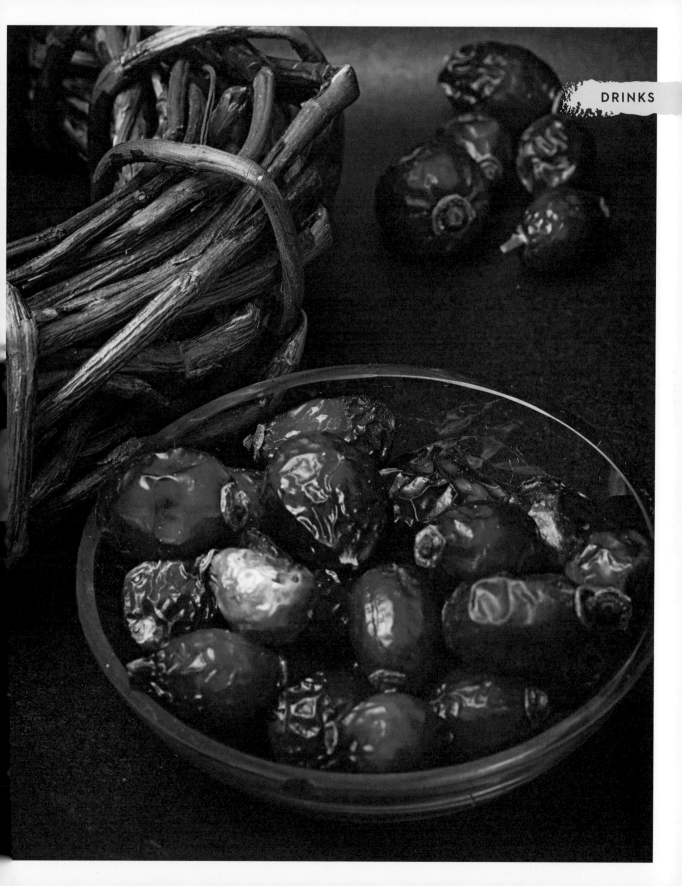

PINK HEART CACAO LATTE

 Heart Health, Gut Health, Blood Sugar Balance, Mood Booster

Not only pretty, this pink latte has absolute superpowers in the antioxidant department. Cacao and beet may not sound like a great combination, but trust me, it works! This beverage protects the heart, improves digestion, supports the blood sugar, and purifies the blood.

INGREDIENTS

1 cup (2.4 dl) hot water

¼ cup (40 g) raw cashews, soaked for at least two hours and rinsed

1 tbsp cacao powder

1½ tspn beet powder

1 tspn schisandra berry powder

½ tspn ground ginger

½ tspn ground cinnamon

1 tspn coconut nectar or maple syrup

DIRECTIONS

1. Place all the ingredients into a high-speed blender and blend for 1 minute or until smooth and creamy. Pour into a mug and enjoy!

·····**MAKES ONE SERVING**

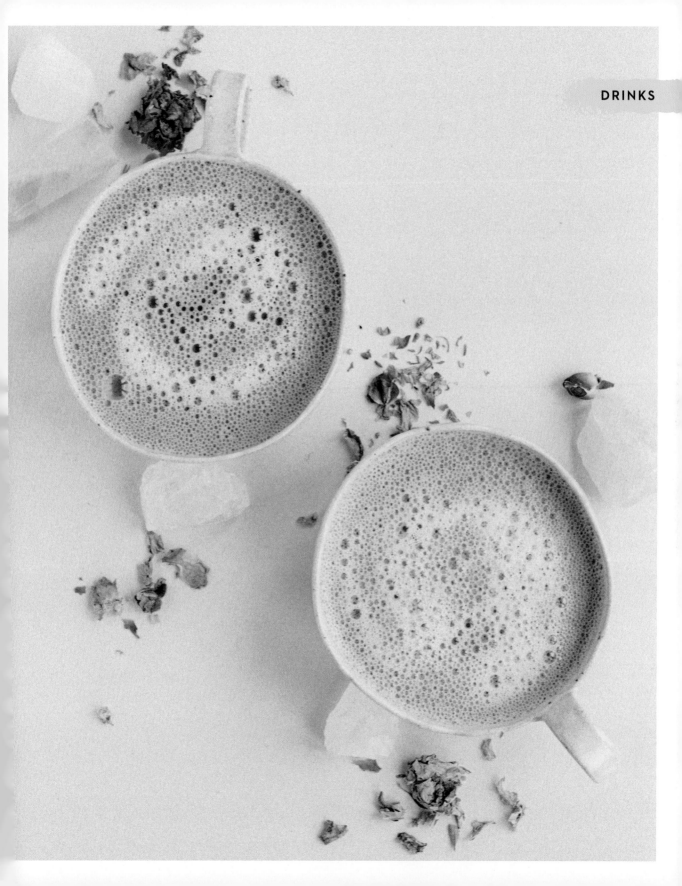

NIGHT-NIGHT MILK

 Restful Sleep, Calming, Beauty Enhancing

Most adaptogens are taken early in the day because they have a
stimulating effect. This mix is perfect to drink right
before bed for a soothing, calming, restful night of sleep.

INGREDIENTS

1 tbsp coconut butter

⅛ tspn ground cardamom

⅛ tspn ground cinnamon

⅛ tspn ground nutmeg

1 Medjool date, pitted

1 cup (2.4 dl) nut milk of your
choice, hot

½ tspn powdered rose petals

⅛ tspn ashwagandha powder

⅛ tspn shatavari powder

⅛ tspn he shou wu powder

⅛ tspn velvet bean powder

DIRECTIONS

1. Place all ingredients in a high-speed blender and blend for
30 seconds or until smooth and creamy. Pour into a mug and enjoy!

MAKES ONE SERVING

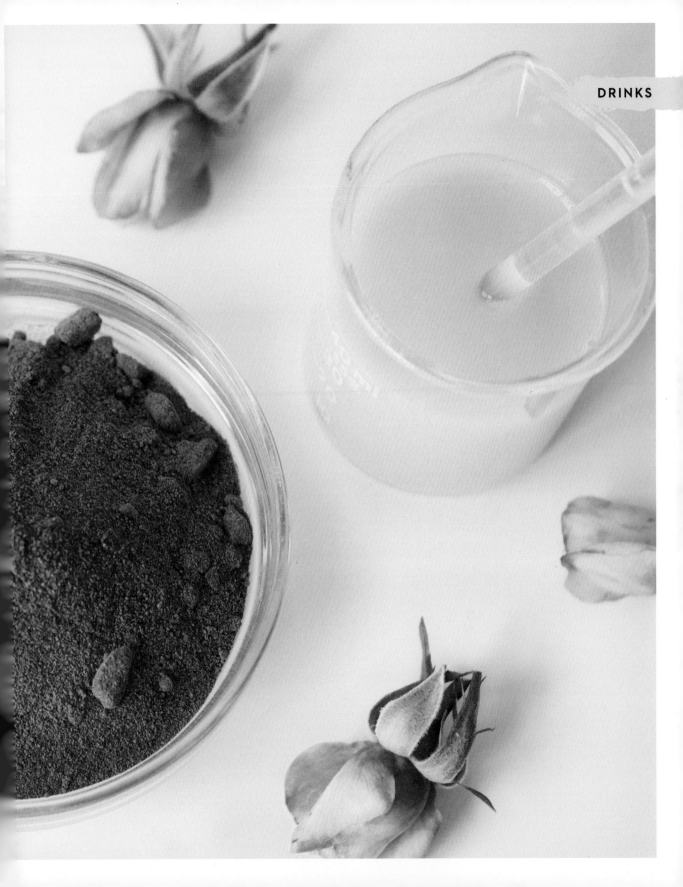

GET-RID-OF-MY-PMS CHAI

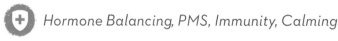 *Hormone Balancing, PMS, Immunity, Calming*

This chai uses the adaptogen suma (Brazilian ginseng), a plant used to balance hormones, treat PMS symptoms, and increase sexual energy. Sip this tea slowly and feel the rewards as your body and mind calm down.

INGREDIENTS

1 cup (2.4 dl) water

½ cup (1.18 dl) unsweetened cashew milk

2 tspn coconut nectar

2 tspn suma root powder

4 cardamom pods, mashed

1 small cinnamon stick

½ inch (1.3 cm) piece ginger root, peeled and sliced

½ tspn fennel seeds

DIRECTIONS

1. Place all ingredients into a medium saucepan over medium heat. Bring to a boil. Turn off the heat, cover, and allow to steep for 5 minutes. Strain into your favorite mug and enjoy!

MAKES ONE SERVING

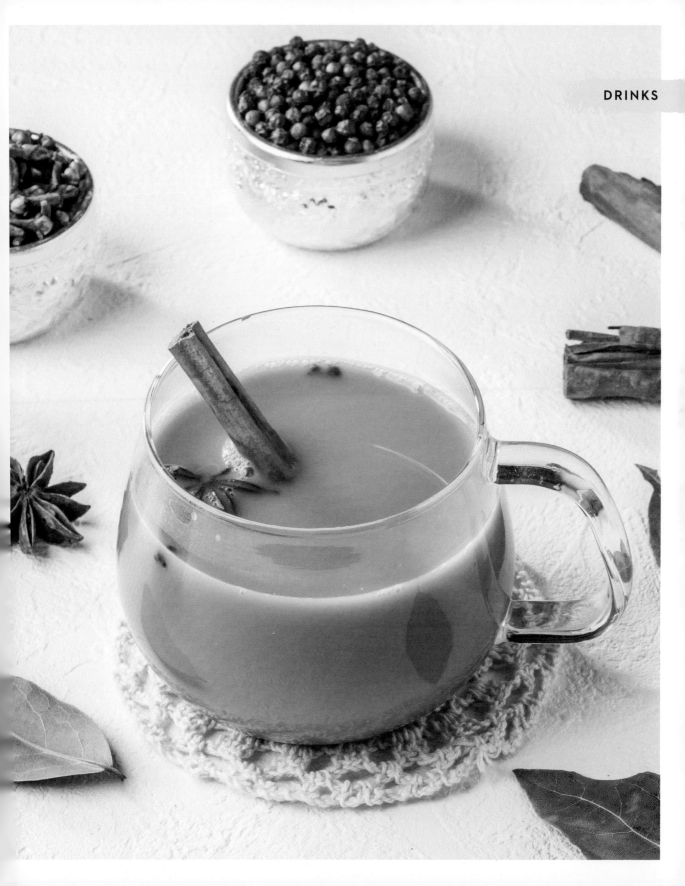

GOLD-STAR LATTE

 Healing, Gut Health, Anti-inflammatory

This beautiful golden latte is comforting—and it's also an incredible anti-inflammatory potion. With the combination of turmeric and baobab, as well as reishi and astragalus, its stress-relieving powers and healing effects are second to none!

INGREDIENTS

1 tbsp almond butter

1 tspn coconut nectar
or maple syrup

2 tspn coconut oil

½ tspn baobab powder

½ tspn astragalus, powdered

½ tspn reishi, powdered

½ tspn ground turmeric

⅛ tspn ground nutmeg

⅛ tspn ground cardamom

⅛ tspn ground cinnamon

⅛ tspn ground cloves

⅛ tspn Himalayan pink sea salt

⅛ tspn freshly ground black
pepper

1 cup (2.4 dl) nut milk of your
choice, hot

DIRECTIONS

1. Combine all ingredients in a high-speed blender and blend for 30 seconds or until smooth and creamy. Pour into a mug and enjoy!

····**MAKES ONE SERVING**

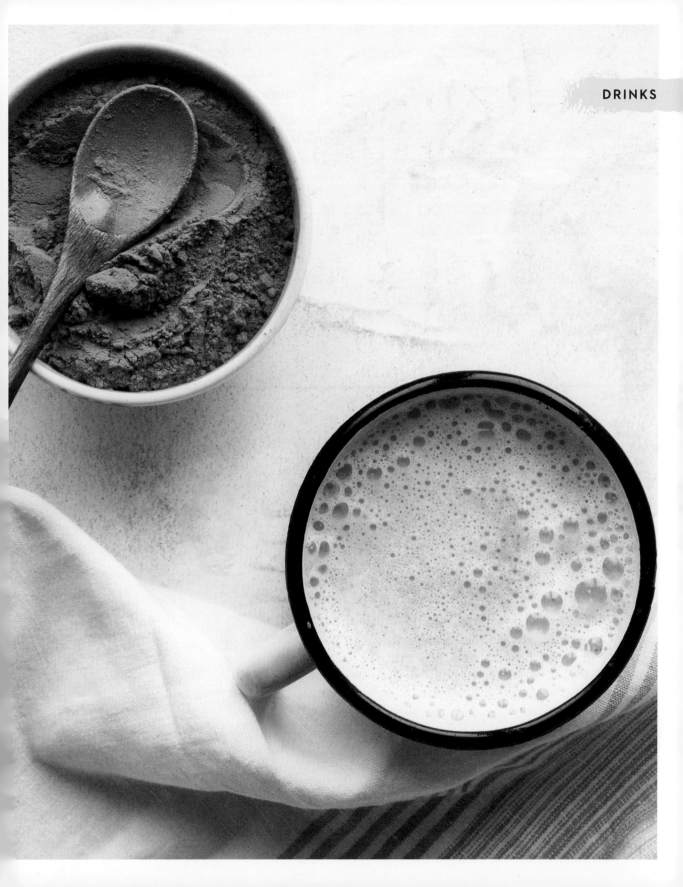

IMMUNE-BOOSTING HOT CHOCOLATE

 Immunity, Aphrodisiac, Hormone Balancer, Energy

Wow, this hot chocolate is decadent and oh so delicious! With mood-boosting chocolate and velvet bean, antioxidants galore, and hormone balance/libido boost from the maca, this drink is sure to be an all-around pleaser.

INGREDIENTS

¼ cup (6 g) raw cashews, soaked for at least two hours, rinsed and drained

1 cup (2.4 dl) water

⅛ tspn Himalayan pink sea salt

¾ cup (95 g) 70% dark chocolate, roughly chopped

1 tspn coconut nectar or maple syrup

¼ tspn ground cinnamon

¼ tspn ashwagandha, powdered

¼ tspn velvet bean, powdered

¼ tspn maca, powdered

1 tspn vanilla extract

DIRECTIONS

1. Combine the soaked cashews, water, and salt in a high-speed blender. Blend on high for one minute or until thick and creamy.

2. Transfer the nut milk to a heavy-bottomed saucepan over medium heat. Add in the chopped chocolate, nectar, or maple syrup cinnamon, ashwagandha, velvet bean, and maca. Whisk to combine and continue whisking until hot and steamy. Do not boil.

3. Pour into a mug and enjoy slowly!

····MAKES ONE SERVING

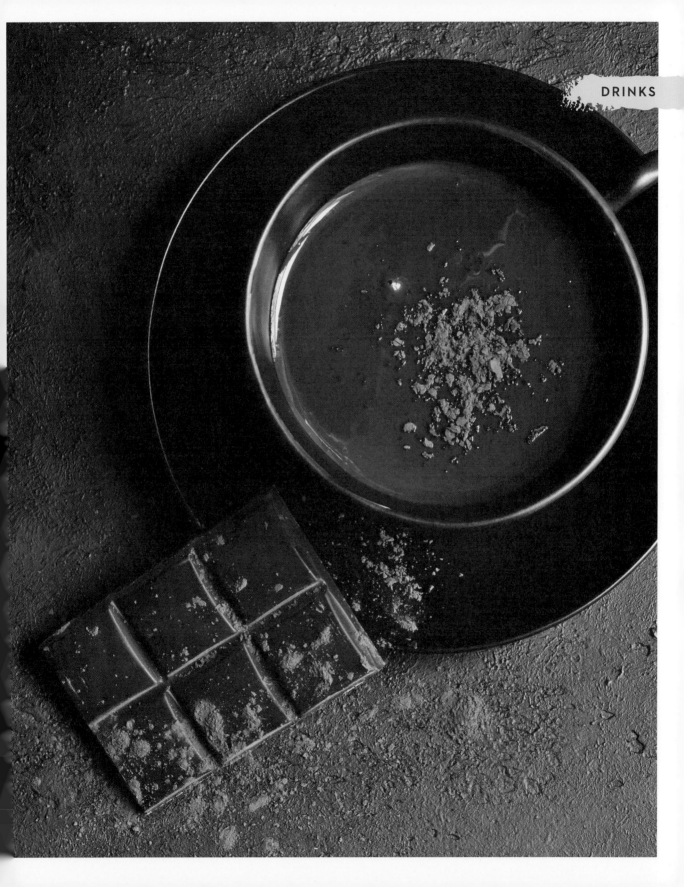

UBER DETOX SMOOTHIE

 Detoxification, Immunity, Antioxidant

This green detox beverage is a powerhouse! With its combination of shilajit resin and chlorella, you'll be helping your body rid itself of heavy metals, toxins, and everyday environmental pollutants.

INGREDIENTS

1 cup (2.4 dl) coconut water

1 cup (165 g) frozen mango chunks

½ cup (132 g) starfruit, peeled and chopped

500 mg shilajit resin

1 tspn chlorella powder

DIRECTIONS

1. Combine all ingredients in a high-powered blender. Blend on high speed for one minute or until smooth and creamy. Enjoy!

MAKES ONE SERVING

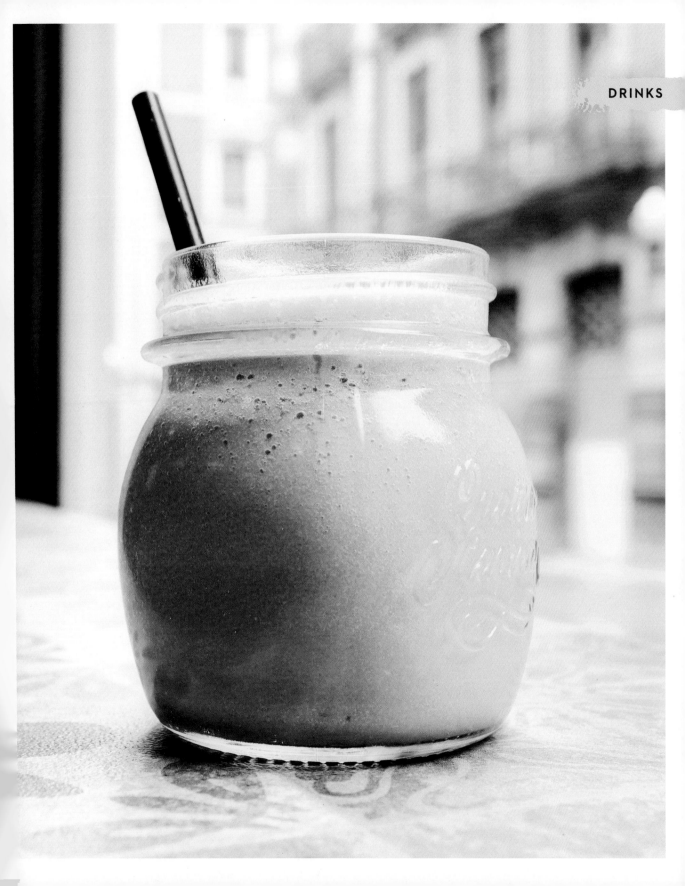

ELECTROLYTE-BETTER THAN YOUR TYPICAL SPORTS DRINK

 Hydration, Energy, Gut Health, Adrenal and Thyroid Function

This is not your average sports drink—it's so much better! A natural
energy booster, electrolyte balancer, digestive health promoter,
and adrenal and thyroid balancer, this drink is a perfect addition to your
sweat session.

INGREDIENTS

¼ cup (0.6 dl) coconut water

1 tspn goji powder

30 drops holy basil extract

¼ tspn schisandra berry powder

¼ tspn rhodiola powder

⅛ tspn Himalayan pink sea salt

¾ cup (1.8 dl) sparkling water

DIRECTIONS

1. Combine the coconut water, goji powder, holy basil, schisandra
berry powder, rhodiola, and sea salt in a large glass. Stir to combine.
Pour in sparkling water and enjoy!

MAKES ONE SERVING

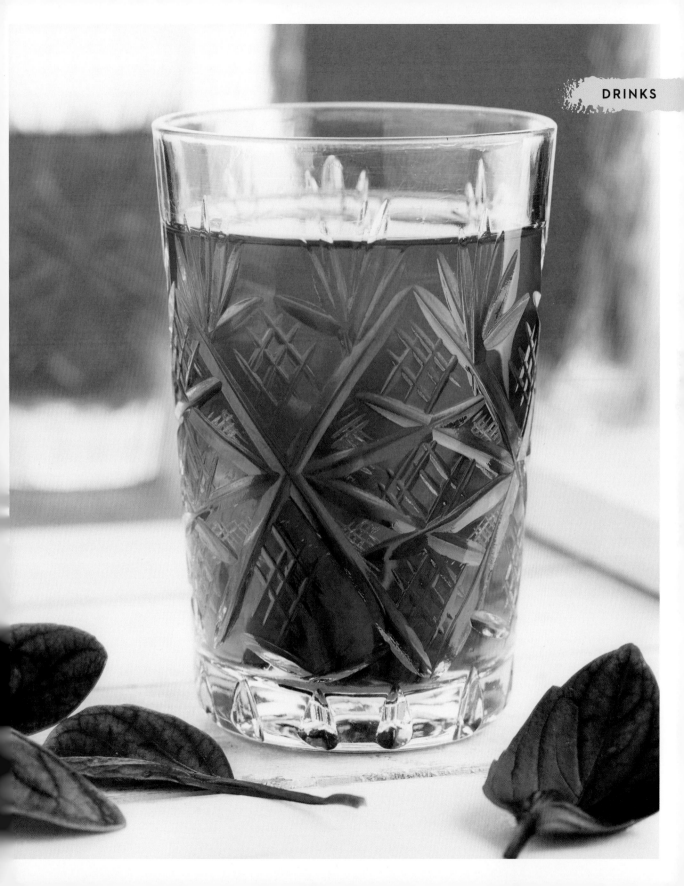

SOOTHE-MY-GRIEF TONIC

 Sadness Remedy, Mood Booster, Immune Booster

Albizia is a natural mood tonic, often used to aid in grief and sadness.
It is a little bitter, but combined with fresh berries or peaches and rose
water, this makes for a soothing drink to calm the spirit.

INGREDIENTS

3 raspberries

2 slices fresh peach

1½ cups (3.5 dl) sparkling water

15 to 30 drops albizia extract

15 to 30 drops rhodiola extract

1 tbsp rose water

Mint leaves, for garnish

DIRECTIONS

1. In the bottom of a large glass, muddle the raspberries and peach
with a muddler.

2. Pour in the sparkling water, albizia extract, rhodiola extract, and
rose water and stir to combine. Enjoy!

MAKES ONE SERVING

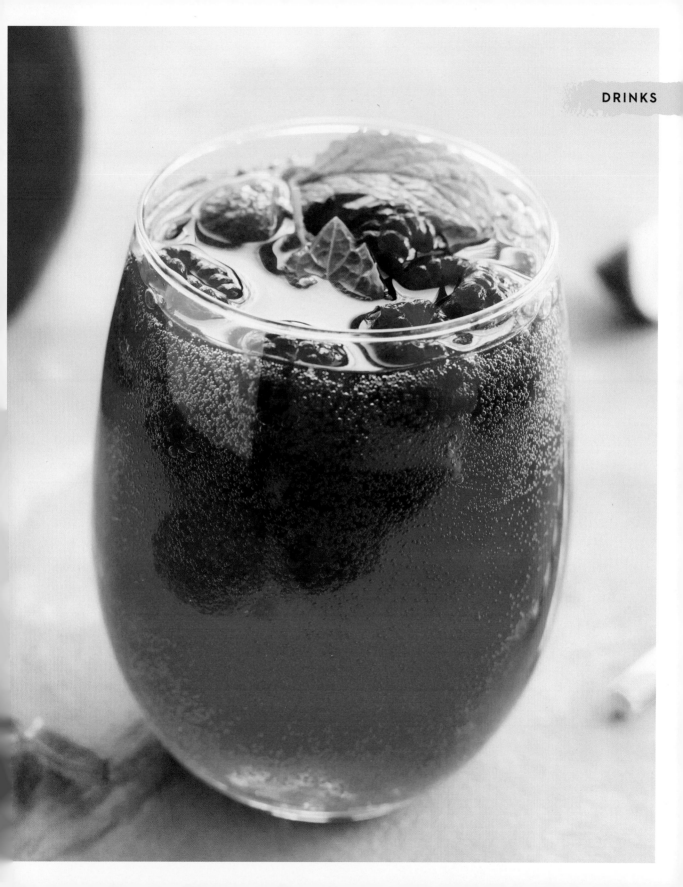

HELP-ME-STUDY TONIC

 Memory, Brain Health, Cognitive Enhancer

This tonic is a must if you need to focus or study for a test. Used in Ayurveda for thousands of years, it's considered excellent to support memory, creativity, motivation, and brain and nerve health.

INGREDIENTS

2 cups (4.7 dl) water

1 bag green tea

1 tspn maple syrup

2 tbsp freshly squeezed lemon juice

½ tspn fresh ginger, peeled and grated

½ tspn fresh turmeric root, peeled and grated

⅛ tspn freshly ground black pepper

⅛ tspn Himalayan pink sea salt

⅛ tspn cayenne pepper

⅛ tspn ashwagandha powder

140 mg bacopa extract or 1 serving of tincture

DIRECTIONS

1. In a small saucepan, bring 1 cup (2.4 dl) water to a boil. Remove from heat and add in the bag of green tea; allow to steep for 2–5 minutes.

2. Remove the tea bag and stir in the maple syrup.

3. Add the mixture to a mason jar with a tight-fitting lid. Add the other cup of cold water and the remaining ingredients. Shake well until fully mixed. Enjoy!

MAKES ONE SERVING

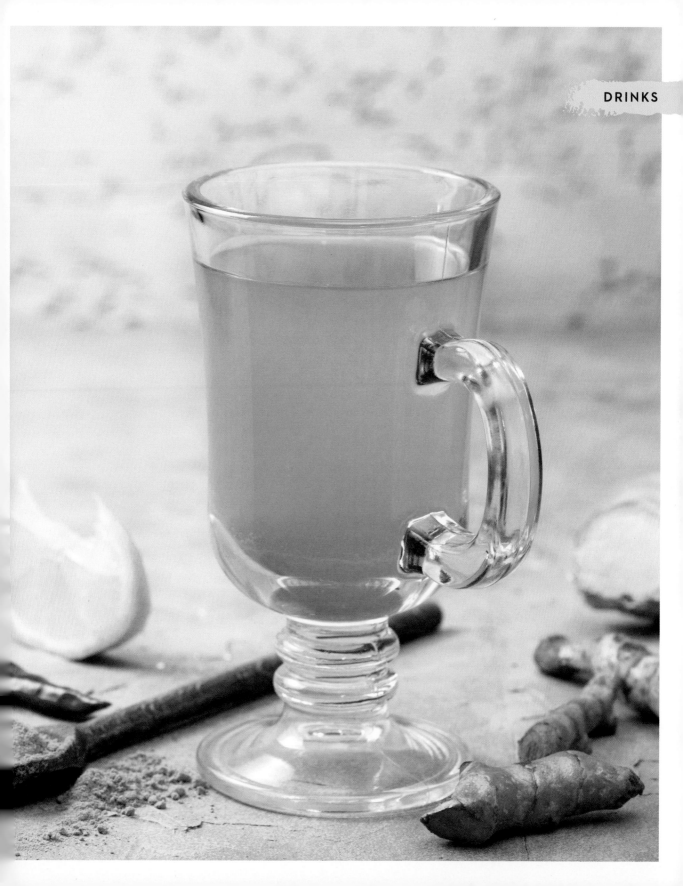

BLUE ANTIOXIDANT LATTE

 Energy, Libido, Beauty, Relaxation

I absolutely love this latte for its color, but its health benefits are wonderful too! Blue spirulina, butterfly pea flower powder, amla, and pine pollen come together with creamy cashews to create a rejuvenating yet relaxing drink that's loaded with antioxidants.

INGREDIENTS

1 cup (2.4 dl) cashew milk

1 tbsp coconut nectar
or maple syrup

½ tspn butterfly pea
flower powder

½ tspn blue spirulina

½ tspn pine pollen

½ tspn amla powder

½ tspn vanilla extract

¼ tspn ground cinnamon

DIRECTIONS

1. In a small, heavy-bottomed pan, add the milk over medium heat and warm until hot (but not boiling). Whisk in the coconut nectar or maple syrup until dissolved.

2. Add the butterfly pea flower powder, blue spirulina, pine pollen, amla, vanilla extract, and cinnamon into a large mug.

3. While whisking, add in the hot cashew milk. Enjoy!

MAKES ONE SERVING

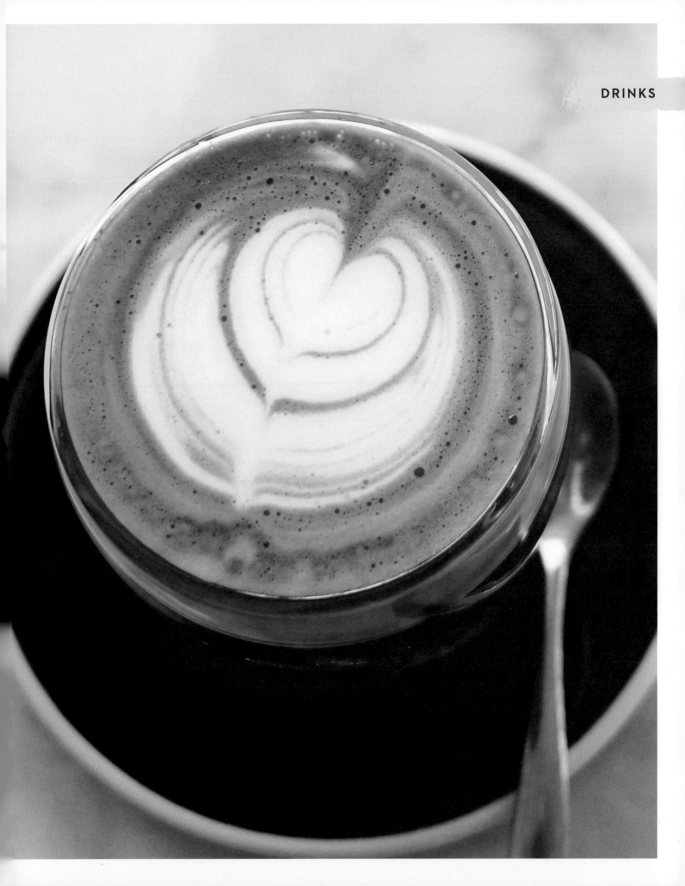

DETOXIFYING TEA

 Liver Detox, Increases Metabolism, Cold and Flu Fighter

This tea is traditionally made by combining guduchi, ashwagandha, and aloe vera. It's known as a whole-body detoxifier, but it also helps ward off colds and flu, increases the metabolism, balances blood sugar, and lowers fevers.

INGREDIENTS

½ cup (1.18 dl) water

½ cup (1.18 dl) aloe vera juice

1 tspn coconut nectar
or maple syrup

½ tspn guduchi powder

½ tspn ashwagandha powder

DIRECTIONS

1. Combine all ingredients in a high-powered blender. Blend on high for one minute or until smooth and creamy. Enjoy!

MAKES ONE SERVING

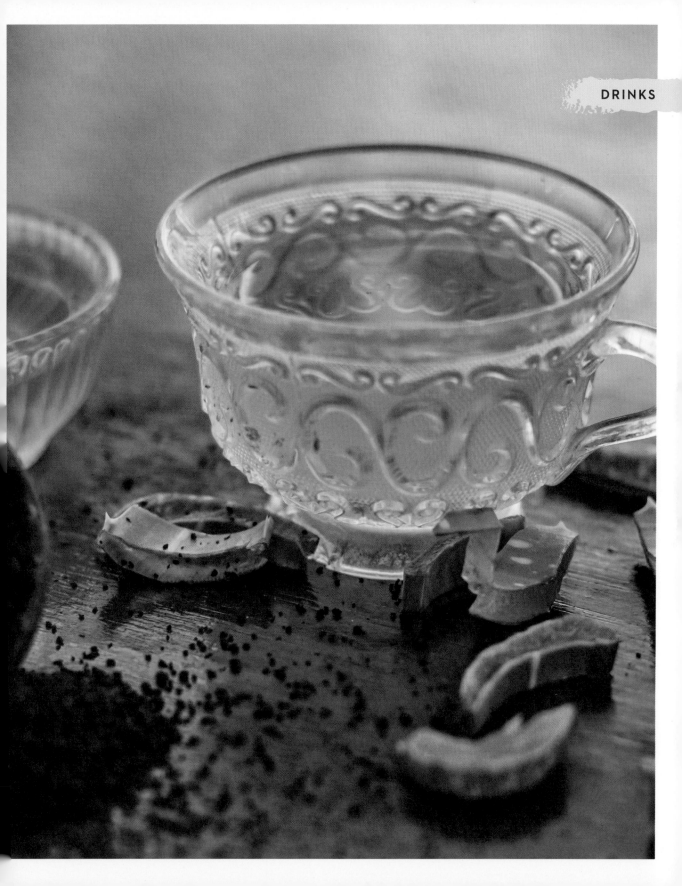

IMMORTALITY-PLEASE TEA

 Homeostasis, Liver Function, Heart Health, Energizing, Longevity, Endurance

Known as "the tea of immortality," this powerful blend of jiaogulan (*Gynostemma pentaphyllum*), shisho, and goji berries is energizing when needed, calming when it's time to relax. You'll feel balanced and energized without feeling jittery! Drink up hot or cold.

INGREDIENTS

1 cup (2.4 dl) water

1 tspn jiaogulan powder

2 shisho leaves

15 dried goji berries

DIRECTIONS

1. In a small saucepan over high heat, add the water and bring to a boil. Add the herbs and allow to steep for 10 minutes. Strain into your favorite mug.

2. Pour over ice or enjoy warm.

MAKES ONE SERVING

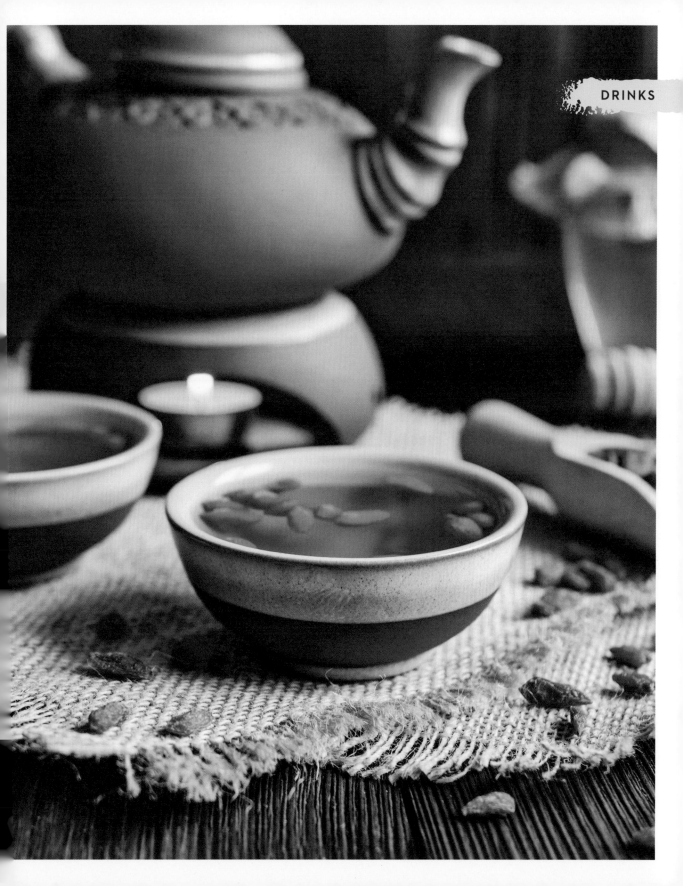

BRAIN BOOST TONIC

 Homeostasis, Focus, Mental Clarity, Energizing

This tonic is a blend of holy basil, gotu kola, ginger, and kombucha. Drink in the morning for a perfect pick-me-up, or in the afternoon, when we get sluggish and need a little energy to make it through the second half of our day.

INGREDIENTS

2 cups (4.7 dl) water

1½ tbsp gotu kola powder

1½ tbsp holy basil powder

1-inch (2.5 cm) fresh ginger, peeled and sliced

2 tspn coconut nectar

1 tspn coconut oil

1 tspn freshly squeezed lemon juice

2 tbsp ginger kombucha

Orange slice, for garnish

Sprig of mint, for garnish

DIRECTIONS

1. In a small saucepan, add the water, gotu kola, and holy basil. Bring to a boil over high heat. Remove from heat and allow to steep for 20 minutes.

2. Strain the herbs from the liquid and pour into a blender.

3. Add the ginger, coconut nectar, coconut oil, and lemon juice. Blend on high speed for one minute or until smooth and creamy.

4. Pour into two glasses, top with kombucha and garnish with a mint sprig and orange slice. Serve and enjoy!

MAKES TWO SERVINGS

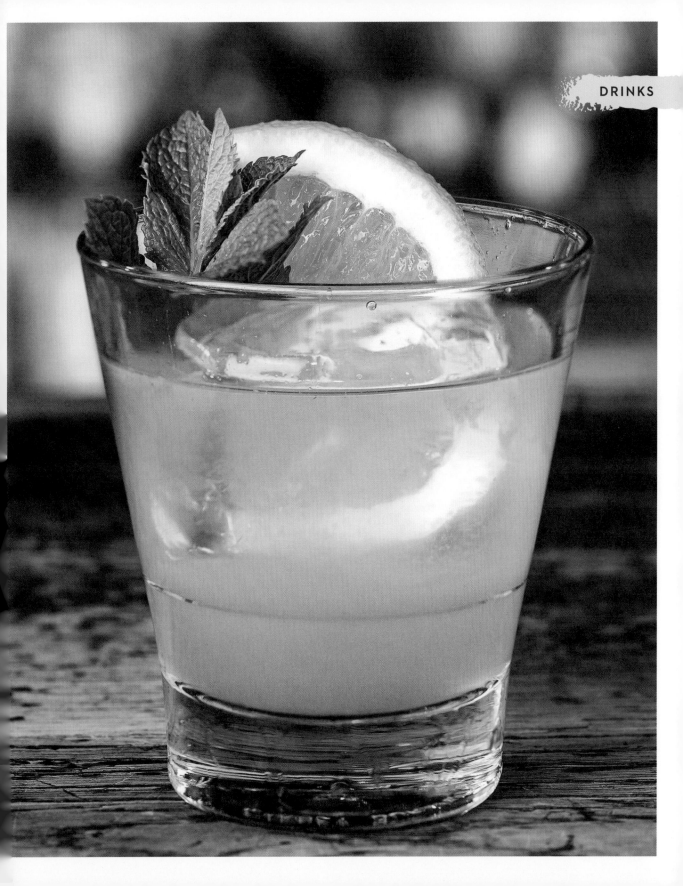

GLOW SMOOTHIE

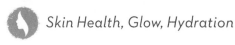 *Skin Health, Glow, Hydration*

This morning smoothie is a perfect start to the day. Loaded with healthy fats, electrolytes, skin-plumping superpowders, and antioxidant-loaded berries, this one is sure to make you glow from within.

INGREDIENTS

1 cup (2.4 dl) coconut water

½ cup (90 g) mix of frozen raspberries, blueberries, and/or strawberries

1 tbsp elderberry extract

1 tspn coconut butter

1 tspn sea buckthorn powder

¼ tspn amla powder

¼ tspn schisandra berry powder

DIRECTIONS

1. Place all ingredients in a high-speed blender. Blend on high for one minute or until smooth and creamy. Pour into a large glass and enjoy!

MAKES ONE SERVING.

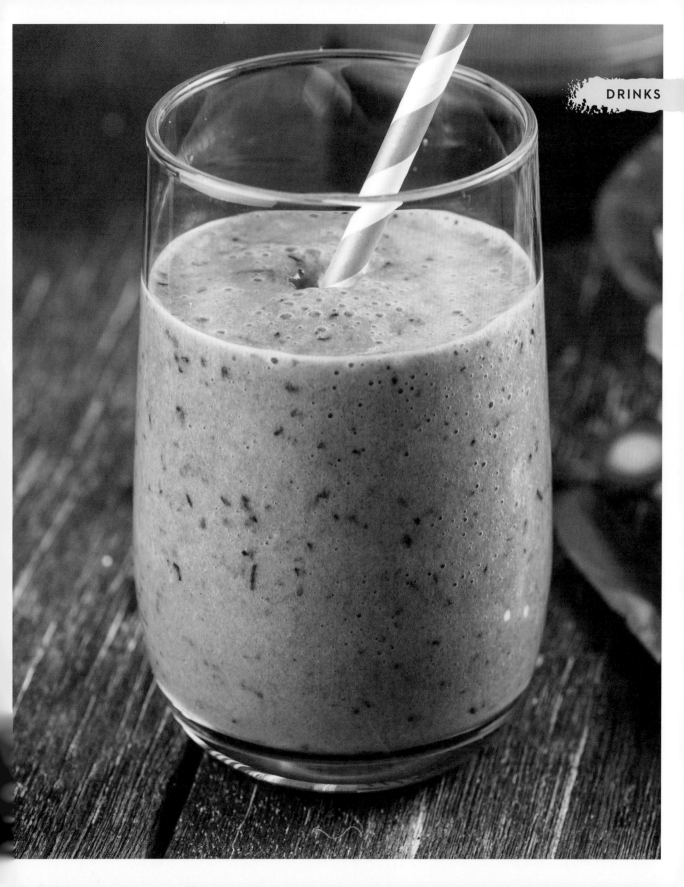

UNDER-THE-WEATHER MISO MUSHROOM SOUP

 Immunity, Anti-inflammatory, Concentration, Strength, Energy

This miso soup is like no other. Comforting, nourishing, nurturing, grounding, healing, and warming, all in one little bowl, its powers are unmatched when it comes to boosting energy and immunity, reducing inflammation, and building strength.

INGREDIENTS

½ ounce dried oyster mushrooms

½ ounce dried porcini mushrooms

½ ounce dried shiitake mushrooms

½ ounce dried maitake mushrooms

2 cups (4.7 dl) boiling water

2 quarts (1.9 l) water

2 sheets kombu

6 cloves garlic, peeled and mashed

3-inches (8 cm) fresh ginger, peeled and sliced

2 sweet onions, peeled and quartered

2 large carrots, peeled and roughly chopped

2 tbsp turmeric powder

1 cup (2.4 dl) organic white miso

2 tbsp reishi powder

2 tbsp cordyceps powder

2 tbsp chaga powder

2 tbsp lion's mane powder

6 scallions, cleaned and thinly sliced

DIRECTIONS

1. Add the dried mushrooms in a large bowl and cover with 2 cups (4.7 dl) boiling water. Allow to sit for 20 minutes. While the mushrooms are soaking, make the broth.

2. In a large stock pot over medium-high heat, add the 2 quarts (1.9 l) water, kombu, garlic, ginger, onions, and carrots. Bring to a boil, then reduce heat to simmer.

3. After the dried mushrooms have soaked, add them to the simmering stock.

4. Using a fine-mesh strainer, strain the mushroom soaking liquid and add it to the broth as well. Continue to simmer the liquid for two hours.

5. Remove the broth from the heat and allow to cool slightly. Strain through a fine-mesh strainer, pressing to release all the flavors, then discard the solids.

6. Add the strained broth back to the stock pot, whisk in the turmeric, miso, mushroom powders, and scallions. Serve hot and enjoy!

MAKES SIX SERVINGS

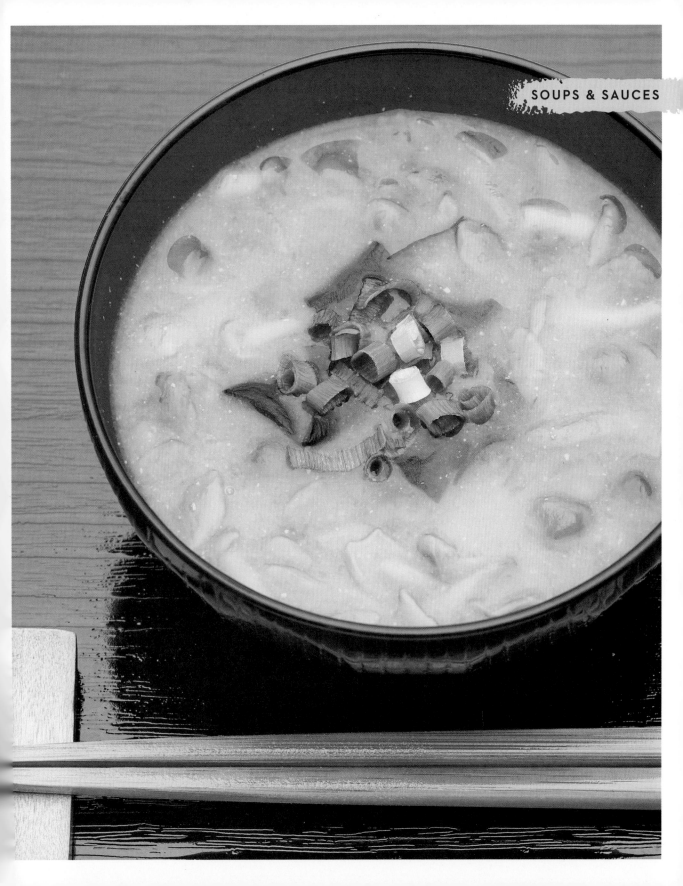

MUSCLE-BUILDING YAM SOUP

 Muscle-building, Strengthening, Immunity, Anti-inflammatory

This soup is hearty, rich, and nourishing. Combining eleuthero, astragalus, ashwagandha, reishi, shiitake, and turmeric gives it muscle-building, strengthening, and anti-inflammatory powers. Include in a meal after a grueling workout to aid in recovery.

INGREDIENTS

3 tbsp coconut oil

1 large sweet onion, diced

4 garlic cloves, minced

3 cups (675 g) purple yam, peeled and cubed

2 tbsp red curry paste

1 tbsp turmeric powder

6 cups (14.2 dl) vegetable stock

2 tbsp astralagus powder

2 tbsp eleuthero powder

2 tbsp ashwagandha powder

2 tbsp reishi mushroom powder

2 tbsp shiitake mushroom powder

1 cup (2.4 dl) coconut cream

¼ cup (15 g) cilantro, chopped

DIRECTIONS

1. Add coconut oil in a large stock pot over medium heat. Once hot, add the onion and sauté for 5 minutes or until tender. Add in the garlic and stir for 30 seconds.

2. Add the cubed yam and sauté for seven to 10 minutes or until the yam begins to soften and is slightly caramelized.

3. Stir in the curry paste and turmeric. Stir for 30 seconds or until fragrant.

4. Add in the vegetable stock, increase the heat to high and bring to a boil. Reduce the heat to a simmer and cook for 30 minutes.

5. Remove from heat. Add in the astralagus, eleuthero, ashwagandha, reishi, shiitake, and coconut cream. Using a burr mixer, puree the soup until creamy or carefully transfer the mixture to a blender and blend until smooth.

6. Ladle into bowls and serve with cilantro. Enjoy!

MAKES SIX TO EIGHT SERVINGS

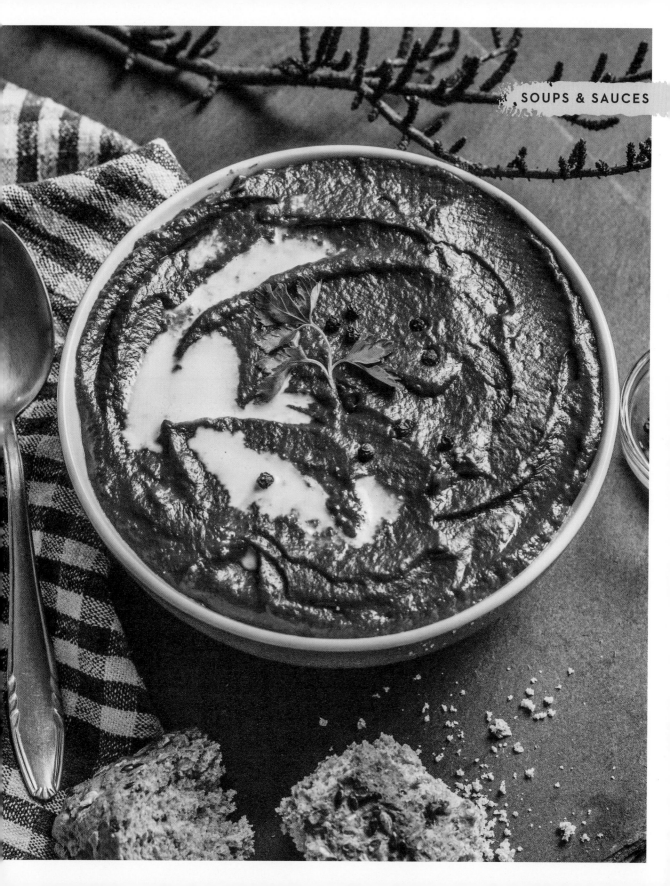

FOCUS-ON-THIS PESTO

 Focus, Concentration, Increase Milk Supply

This is one for vegans, breastfeeding mothers, and students alike!
Ashitaba is a nutrient-dense green vegetable that's perfect when paired
with basil, nutritional yeast, and macadamia for this delightful vitamin
B6- and B12-packed pesto. Ashitaba is not easy to find fresh, but growing
it is super easy and well worth the effort!

INGREDIENTS

1 cup (125 g) raw macadamias, soaked for 2 hours and rinsed

4 garlic cloves, peeled

1 cup (2.4 dl) nutritional yeast

1 cup (20 g) fresh ashitaba leaves, washed and dried

1 cup (20 g) fresh basil leaves, washed and dried

1½ tspn Himalayan pink sea salt

1 tspn freshly ground black pepper

½ cup (1.18 dl) extra virgin olive oil

DIRECTIONS

1. In the bowl of a food processor, combine the soaked macadamias, garlic, nutritional yeast, ashitaba, basil leaves, salt, and pepper. Pulse until roughly chopped, about 20 to 25 times.

2. Scrape down the sides, put the lid back on and turn the machine on low. Slowly add in the olive oil until well combined. Enjoy with pasta, tofu, or anything else your heart desires.

----**MAKES ONE AND A HALF CUPS**

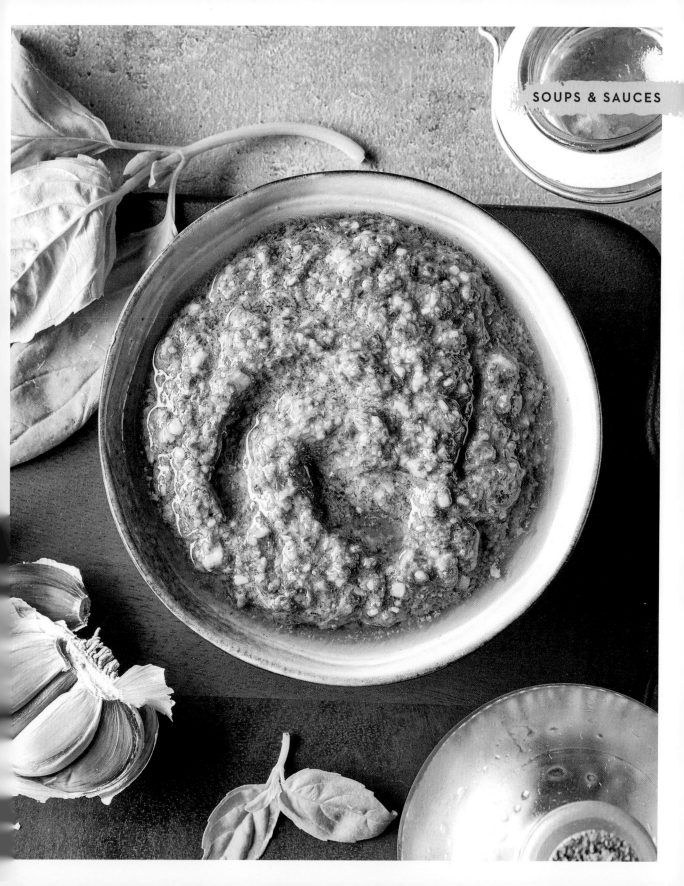

GOOD-FOR-MY-GUT
WALNUT SPREAD

 Gut Health, Digestion, Treatment of Psoriasis and Eczema

This homemade walnut spread uses burdock root powder and hawthorn berry powder to make it extra special. It's great on toast, pancakes, waffles, or used any other way you'd like. Burdock is especially great if you've been on antibiotics: it helps restore the gut back to homeostasis.

INGREDIENTS

1 cup (125 g) sprouted walnuts

2 tspn maple syrup

1½ tspn burdock root powder

1 tspn hawthorn berry powder

½ tspn ground cinnamon

½ tspn Himalayan pink sea salt

⅛ tspn ground cardamom

DIRECTIONS

1. Add the walnuts to the bowl of a food processor and pulse eight to ten times to break the walnuts down into smaller pieces.

2. Add in the maple syrup, burdock, hawthorn berry, cinnamon, sea salt, and cardamom and blend on high for 3–5 minutes or until the mixture resembles a nut butter. You may need to stop and scrape down the sides from time to time.

3. Keep in an airtight glass container and enjoy! Will keep for three to five days.

----MAKES ONE CUP

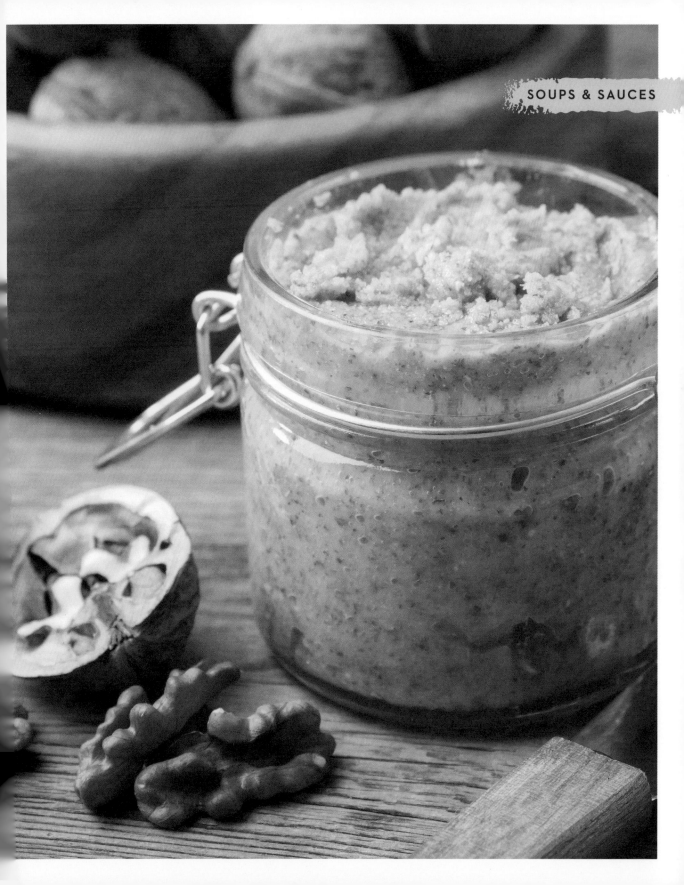

SUPPORT-MY-SYSTEM SEASONING

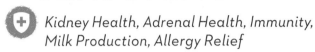 *Kidney Health, Adrenal Health, Immunity, Milk Production, Allergy Relief*

This fabulous, all-purpose seasoning uses nettle seeds and dried leaves from the plant, both of which are easy to find online. Use this seasoning on roasted vegetables, in soups, in stews, or as a substitute for boring old salt!

INGREDIENTS

½ cup (10 g) dried nettle leaves, ground

½ cup (65 g) nettle seeds

¼ cup (66 g) Himalayan pink sea salt

1 tbsp dried thyme, powdered

1 tbsp dried basil, powdered

1 tbsp dried parsley, powdered

1 tbsp garlic powder

1 tbsp onion powder

DIRECTIONS

1. Mix all ingredients in a medium bowl. Store in an airtight container in a cool, dark place. Enjoy!

MAKES TWO CUPS

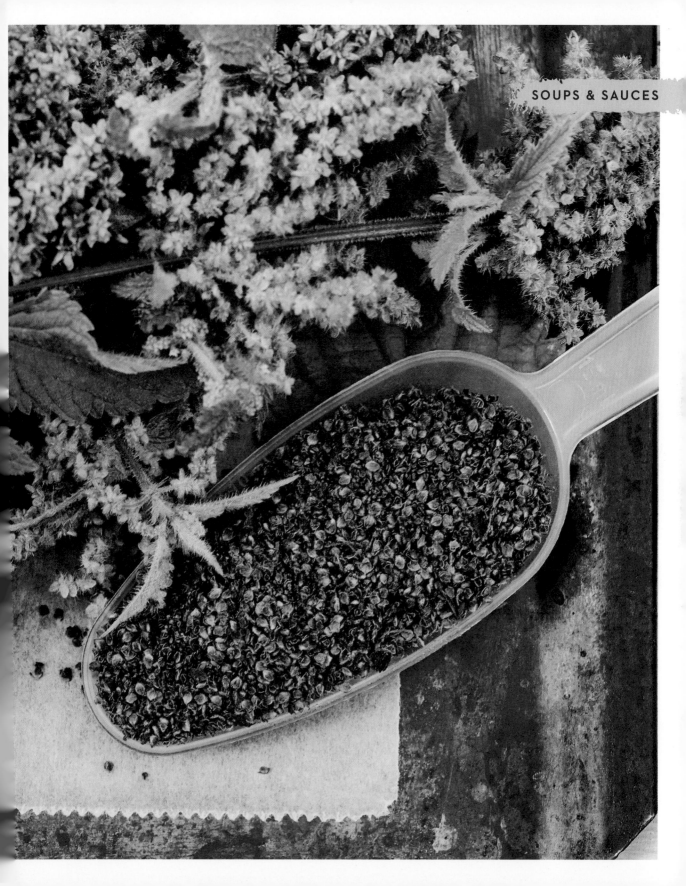

ENERGY-BOOST CHIA PUDDING

 Energy Booster, Immune Support, Athletic Performance

This chia pudding is a great way to start the day, whether going for a long workout or into a long workday. It uses American ginseng tea bags steeped in almond milk for the base, as well as powdered American ginseng. The extra step is more time consuming but making this pudding the night before ensures an easy and energizing to-go breakfast!

INGREDIENTS

Pudding

1 cup (2.4 dl) unsweetened vanilla almond milk

2 American ginseng tea bags

¼ cup (32 g) organic chia seeds

1 tspn maple syrup

½ tspn American ginseng powder

¼ tspn ground cinnamon

¼ tspn ground cardamom

¼ cup (65 g) coconut yogurt

Topping

1 tbsp maple syrup

4 tbsp pomegranate arils

4 tbsp roasted pistachios, crushed

DIRECTIONS

1. In a small saucepan, add the almond milk over medium heat and bring to a simmer. Turn off the heat, add the tea bags, cover, and let steep for 10 minutes. Squeeze all the liquid from the tea bags, remove, and discard them.

2. Divide the chia seeds into two small mason jars with tight-fitting lids. Add half the steeped milk to each mason jar. Divide the maple syrup, ginseng powder, cinnamon, and cardamom between the two; cover, shake, then allow to marinate in the refrigerator overnight.

3. In the morning, remove the chia puddings from the refrigerator, fold in the coconut yogurt and top each one with half of the toppings. Enjoy!

····**MAKES TWO SERVINGS**

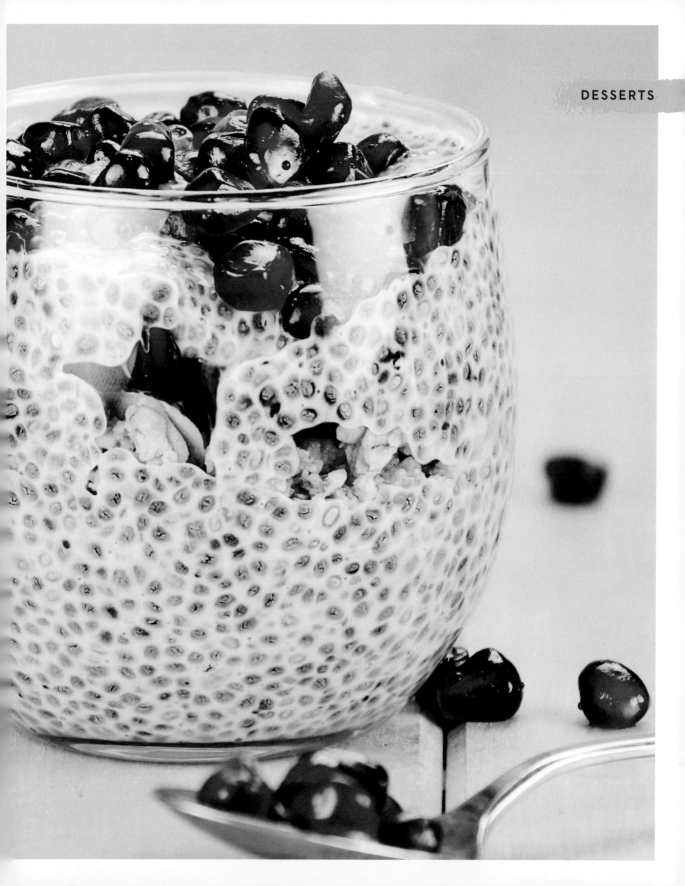

LOVER CHOCOLATE ASIAN GINSENG TRUFFLES

 Aphrodisiac, Male and Female Libido Enhancer, Heart Health

These truffles are a great Valentine's Day treat or just an energizing treat for any day! They're packed with antioxidants, healthy fats, and Asian ginseng powder. The flavor is sweet, earthy, and rich.

INGREDIENTS

Truffles

1 cup (109 g) raw pecans

1 cup (125 g) raw walnuts

10 whole Medjool dates, pitted

1 tbsp cacoa powder

½ tspn ground cinnamon

1 tbsp Asian ginseng root powder

1 tspn maca powder

1¼ cups (130 g) 70% or higher dairy-free dark chocolate, roughly chopped

1½ tspn coconut oil

Toppings

¼ cup (120 g) cocoa nibs, crushed

¼ cup (125 g) walnuts, crushed

¼ tspn Himalayan pink sea salt

DIRECTIONS

1. In the bowl of a food processor, add the pecans and walnuts and blend on high for 1–2 minutes or until finely chopped. Remove and set aside in a large bowl.

2. In the bowl of the same food processor, add the dates and process on high until they are finely chopped and pull away from the sides to form a ball, about 1 minute.

3. Add in the cocoa powder, cinnamon, ginseng powder, maca powder, and half of the reserved chopped nuts. Pulse until the mixture combines and then add in the rest of the nut meal until a dough has formed.

4. Using a small cookie scoop, scoop the dough and roll into balls. Using wet hands, shape and mold each ball, then place each onto a parchment-lined baking sheet. Transfer the balls to the freezer while you prepare the chocolate.

5. In a double boiler, add the chocolate and coconut oil and stir until melted. Be careful not to overheat. Once melted, remove from the heat.

6. Remove the truffles from the freezer and, one at a time, dip into the melted chocolate mixture. Use a fork to tap away any excess chocolate. Transfer the balls back onto the parchment paper and sprinkle with the crushed cocoa nibs, walnuts, and sea salt.

7. Enjoy! Store any leftover truffles in an airtight container at room temperature. You may freeze them if needed, but I doubt they will be around that long.

MAKES FOURTEEN TRUFFLES

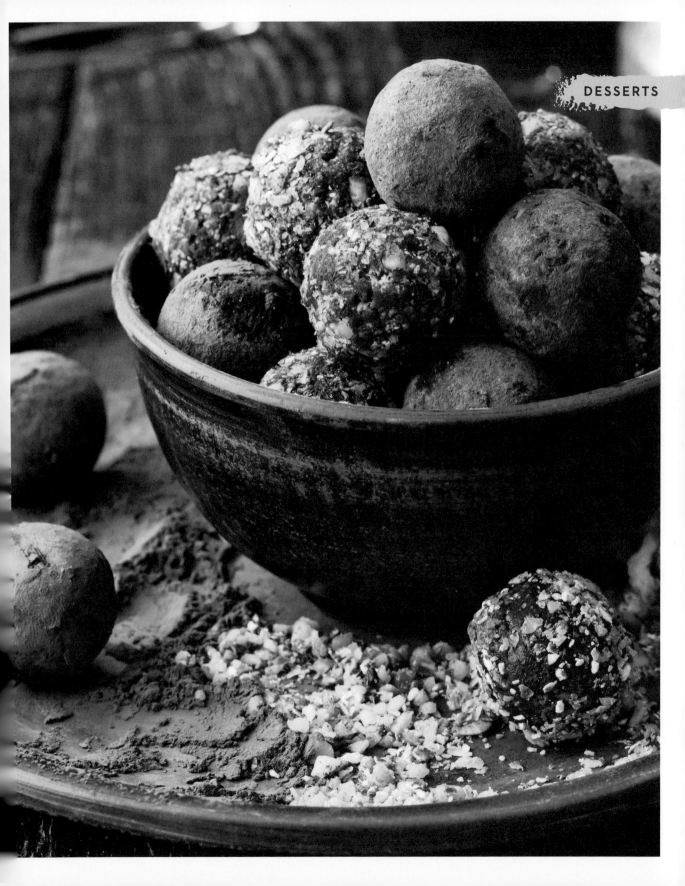

ENHANCE MY ATHLETIC PERFORMANCE TRUFFLES

 Energizing, Cell Growth, Endurance, Recovery

These truffles are a powerful combination of ashwagandha, cordyceps, rhaponticum, and rhodiola. They're designed to help an athlete perform at his or her peak, gain incredible stamina and endurance, and recover at an optimal rate.

INGREDIENTS

Truffles

¼ cup (0.6 dl) coconut oil

½ cup (118 g) raw cocoa powder

¼ cup (0.6 dl) maple syrup

½ tspn Himalayan pink sea salt

¼ tspn ashwagandha powder

¼ tspn cordyceps powder

¼ tspn rhaponticum powder

¼ tspn rhodiola rosea powder

1 tbsp almond or cashew milk

Toppings

2 tbsp cacao nibs, crushed

2 tbsp freeze-dried raspberries, crushed

DIRECTIONS

1. In a small saucepan, warm the coconut oil until just melted. Transfer to a medium bowl.

2. Add the cocoa powder, maple syrup, salt, and all adaptogen powders. Stir to combine.

3. Add in the nut milk. Transfer the mixture to the refrigerator and chill, covered, for 10 minutes.

4. With wet hands, roll the sticky mixture into 12 balls, then roll in the toppings.

5. Place on a parchment-lined tray and transfer to the refrigerator for at least 20 minutes before eating. Enjoy!

····MAKES TWELVE

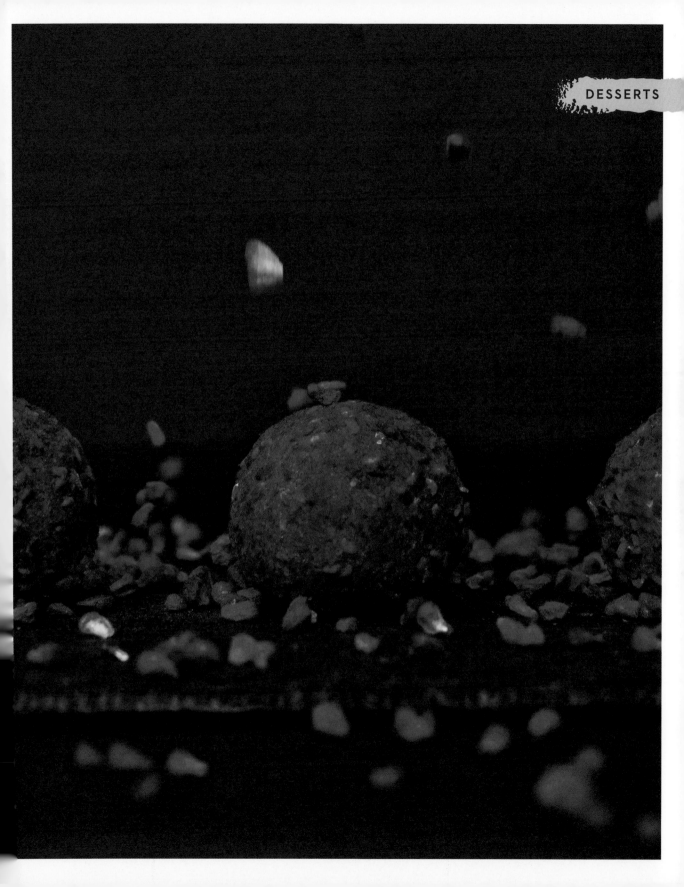

WORKS CITED

1. Firenzuoli F., Gori L., Lombardo G. [The Medicinal Mushroom *Agaricus blazei* Murrill: Review of Literature and Pharmaco-Toxicological Problems.] *Evidence Based Complement Alternative Medicine.* 2008. doi:10.1093/ecam/nem007

2. Ohno S., Sumiyoshi Y., Hashine K., Shirato A., Kyo S., Inoue M. [Phase I Clinical Study of the Dietary Supplement, *Agaricus blazei* Murill, in Cancer Patients in Remission.] *Evidence Based Complement Alternative Medicine.* 2011. doi:10.1155/2011/192381

3. Abdul Manap A.S., Vijayabalan S., Madhavan P., et al. [*Bacopa monnieri*, a Neuroprotective Lead in Alzheimer Disease: A Review on Its Properties, Mechanisms of Action, and Preclinical and Clinical Studies.] *Drug Target Insights.* July 31, 2019. doi:10.1177/1177392819866412

4. Farooqui A.A., Farooqui T., Madan A., Ong J.H., Ong W.Y. [Ayurvedic Medicine for the Treatment of Dementia: Mechanistic Aspects.] *Evidence Based Complement Alternative Medicine.* May 15, 2018. doi:10.1155/2018/2481076

5. Gordon M., Bihari B., Goosby E., Gorter R., Greco M., Guralnik M., Mimura T., Rudinicki V., Wong R., Kaneko Y. [A placebo-controlled trial of the immune modulator, lentinan, in HIV-positive patients: a phase I/II trial.] *AIDS Activities Division, San Francisco General Hospital, CA, USA.* May-June 1998. PMID: 10503166

6. Lampariello L.R., Cortelazzo A., Guerranti R., Sticozzi C., Valacchi G. [The Magic Velvet Bean of *Mucuna pruriens.*] *Traditional Complement Medicine.* 2012. doi:10.1016/s2225-4110(16)30119-5

7. Rijntjes, Michel, Hélio. Teive. [Knowing Your Beans in Parkinson's Disease: A Critical Assessment of Current Knowledge about Different Beans and Their Compounds in the Treatment of Parkinson's Disease and in Animal Models.] *Traditional Complement Medicine.* October 30, 2019. Article ID 1349509.

8. Johns Hopkins University. [American Ginseng to Improve HIV-Associated Fatigue: A Randomized, Placebo-Controlled, Parallel Design, Multiple-Dose Clinical Trial.] *National Center for Complementary and Integrative Health (NCCIH).* June 2018. ClinicalTrials.gov Identifier: NCT01500096. Other Study ID Numbers: NA_00071671

9. Darbinyan V., Kteyan A., Panossian A., Gabrielian E., Wikman G., and Wagner H. [*Rhodiola rosea* in stress induced fatigue–A double blind cross-over study of a standardized extract SHR-5 with a repeated low-dose regimen on the mental performance of healthy physicians during night duty.] *Department of Neurology, Armenian State Medical University, Yerevan, Armenia/Guelbenkian Research Laboratory of Armenian Drug and Medical Technology Agency, Yerevan, Armenia. Swedish Herbal Institute, Gothenburg, Sweden. Institute of Pharmacy, Pharmaceutical Biology, Ludwig Maximilian University, Munich, Germany.* 2000. Phytomedicine, Vol. 7(5), pp. 365–371

10. Fursova A., Gesarevich O., Gonchar A., Trofimova N., Kolosova N. [Dietary supplementation with bilberry extract prevents macular degeneration and cataracts in senesce-accelerated OXYS rats.] *Advanced Gerontol.* 2005. PMID: 16075680

BIBLIOGRAPHY

Chesak, Jennifer. (13 October 2017) *The No BS Guide to Adaptogens for Hormonal Balance and Stress.* Healthline.
healthline.com/health/stress smart-girls-guide-to-adaptogens

Guthrie, Catherine. (January/February 2014) *Ancient Healers: Adaptogens Life.* Time.
experiencelife.com/article/ancient-healers-adaptogens/

Liao, Lian-Ying. (16 November 2018) *A Preliminary Review of Studies on Adaptogens: Comparison of their Bioactivity in TCM with that of Ginseng-Like Herbs Used Worldwide.* Biomed Central.
ncbi.nlm.nih.gov/pmc/articles/PMC6240259/

Noveille, Agatha. (2018) *The Complete Guide to Adaptogens,* Avon, Massachusetts. Simon & Schuster, Inc.

Ratini, Melinda, DO, MS. (15 March 2019) *What is Traditional Chinese Medicine?* WebMD.
webmd.com/balance/guide/what-is-traditional-chinese-medicine#2

Ratini, Melinda, DO, MS. (20 March 2019) *What is Ayurveda?* WebMD
webmd.com/balance/guide/ayurvedic-treatments#1

Time. (28 February 2018) *What are Adaptogens and Why Are People Taking Them?* Time USA, LLC.
time.com/5025278/adaptogens-herbs-stress-anxiety/

Van Wyk, Katrine. (2019) *Super Powders.* New York, New York. W.W. Norton & Company, Inc.

Yance, Donald. (2013) *Adaptogens in Medical Herbalism.* Rochester, Vermont. Healing Arts Press.

Yance, Donald R. Jr. (2000) *Adaptogens: New Conceptions and Uses, Personal Insights and Recent Advances.* Healing Base.
healingbase.com/adaptogens-new-conceptions-and-uses-personal-insights-and-recent-advances/

INDEX

T

V

W